theclinics.com

RHEUMATIC DISEASE CLINICS OF NORTH AMERICA

Osteoporosis

GUEST EDITOR
Philip N. Sambrook, MD

November 2006 • Volume 32 • Number 4

SAUNDERS

An Imprint of Elsevier, Inc.
PHILADELPHIA   LONDON   TORONTO   MONTREAL   SYDNEY   TOKYO

W.B. SAUNDERS COMPANY
A Division of Elsevier Inc.

1600 John F. Kennedy Boulevard • Suite 1800 • Philadelphia, Pennsylvania 19103-2899

http://www.theclinics.com

RHEUMATIC DISEASE   Volume 32, Number
CLINICS OF NORTH AMERICA   ISSN 0889-857
November 2006   ISBN 1-4160-3904-
Editor: Rachel Glover

The ideas and opinions expressed in *Rheumatic Disease Clinics of North America* do not necessarily reflec
those of the Publisher. The Publisher does not assume any responsibility for any injury and/or damag
to persons or property arising out of or related to any use of the material contained in this periodica
The reader is advised to check the appropriate medical literature and the product information current\
provided by the manufacturer of each drug to be administered to verify the dosage, the method and dur;
tion of administration, or contraindications. It is the responsibility of the treating physician or other healt
care professional, relying on independent experience and knowledge of the patient, to determine dru
dosages and the best treatment of the patient. Mention of any product in this issue should not be construe
as endorsement by the contributors, editors, or the Publisher of the product or manufacturers' claims.

Rheumatic Disease Clinics of North America (ISSN 0889-857X) is published quarterly by Elsevier Inc., 360 Par
Avenue South, New York, NY 10010-1710. Months of issue are February, May, August, and Novembe
Business and editorial offices: 1600 John F. Kennedy Boulevard, Suite 1800, Philadelphia, PA 19103-289
Customer Service offices: 6277 Sea Harbor Drive, Orlando, FL 32887-4800. Periodicals postage paid ;
New York, NY and additional mailing offices. Subscription prices are USD 205 per year for US individual;
USD 336 per year for US institutions, USD 103 per year for US students and residents, USD 243 per year fc
Canadian individuals, USD 407 per year for Canadian institutions, USD 270 per year for international ir
dividuals, USD 407 per year for international institutions and USD 135 per year for Canadian and foreig
students/residents. To receive student/resident rate, orders must be accompanied by name of affiliated ir
stitution, date of term, and the *signature* of program/residency coordinator on institution letterhea(
Orders will be billed at individual rate until proof of status received. Foreign air speed delivery is include
in all *Clinics* subscription prices. All prices are subject to change without notice. POSTMASTER: Send a(
dress changes to *Rheumatic Disease Clinics of North America,* Elsevier Periodicals Customer Service, 6277 S∈
Harbor Drive, Orlando, FL 32887-4800. **Customer Service: 1-800-654-2452 (USA). From outside of th**
USA, call (+1) 407-345-4000. E-mail: hhspcs@harcourt.com.

Reprints. For copies of 100 or more of articles in this publication, please contact the Commercial Reprin
Department, Elsevier Inc., 360 Park Avenue South, New York, New York, 10010-1710; Tel.: (+1) 212-63.
3813, Fax: (+1) 212-462-1935, and E-mail: reprints@elsevier.com.

Rheumatic Disease Clinics of North America is covered in *Index Medicus, Current Contents/Clinical Medicin*
Science Citation Index, ISI/BIOMED, and *EMBASE/Excerpta Medica.*

Printed in the United States of America.

GUEST EDITOR

PHILIP N. SAMBROOK, MD, Professor of Rheumatology, Institute of Bone & Joint Research, Royal North Shore Hospital, St. Leonards, Sydney, Australia

CONTRIBUTORS

OMAR M.E. ALBAGHA, MSc, PhD, Lecturer in the Genetic Basis of Bone Disease, Rheumatology Section, Molecular Medicine Centre, University of Edinburgh School of Molecular and Clinical Medicine, Edinburgh, United Kingdom

GEROLAMO BIANCHI, MD, Director, Rheumatology Unit, La Colletta Hospital, Arenzano, Genova, Italy

CYRUS COOPER, DM, FRCP, FMedSci, Professor, Department of Rheumatology, MRC Epidemiology Resource Centre, Southampton General Hospital, Southampton, United Kingdom

ELAINE DENNISON, MB, BChir, MA, MRCP, PhD, Reader, Department of Rheumatology, MRC Epidemiology Resource Centre, Southampton General Hospital, Southampton, United Kingdom

JEAN-PIERRE DEVOGELAER, MD, Clinical Professor of Rheumatology, Department of Medicine, Arthritis Unit, Saint-Luc University Hospital, Université catholique de Louvain, Brussels, Belgium

MATTHEW T. GILLESPIE, PhD, Director, Bone Biology Program, St. Vincent's Institute, Fitzroy, Australia

GIUSEPPE GIRASOLE, MD, PhD, Bone Metabolic Unit, Department of Rheumatology, La Colletta Hospital, Arenzano, Genova, Italy

KENDAL L. HAMANN, MD, Fellow, Division of Endocrinology, Clinical Nutrition, and Vascular Medicine, University of California Davis Medical Center, Sacramento; Sacramento Mather Veterans' Affairs Medical Center, Mather, California

MARC C. HOCHBERG, MD, MPH, Professor of Medicine and Head, Division of Rheumatology, Department of Medicine and Department of Epidemiology and Preventive Medicine, University of Maryland School of Medicine; Maryland Veterans Affairs Health Care System, Baltimore, Maryland

NANCY E. LANE, MD, Professor, Department of Medicine, University of California Davis Medical Center; Director, University of California Davis Center for Healthy Aging, University of California Davis Medical Center, Sacramento, California

MAYSAM ABDIN MOHAMED, MB, BS, MRCP, Specialist Registrar, Department of Rheumatology, Southampton General Hospital, Southampton, United Kingdom

STUART H. RALSTON, MD, FRCP, ARC Professor of Rheumatology, Rheumatology Section, Molecular Medicine Centre, University of Edinburgh School of Molecular and Clinical Medicine, Edinburgh, United Kingdom

IAN R. REID, MD, Professor of Medicine, Faculty of Medical and Health Sciences, University of Auckland, Auckland, New Zealand

EVANGE ROMAS, MD, FRACP, PhD, Director, Rheumatology Research Unit, The University of Melbourne, St. Vincent's Hospital, Fitzroy, Australia

STUART SILVERMAN, MD, FACP, FACR, Clinical Professor of Medicine and Rheumatology, Department of Medicine, Division of Rheumatology, Cedars-Sinai Medical Center/UCLA, The Osteoporosis Medical Center, Beverly Hills, California

LUIGI SINIGAGLIA, MD, Director, Rheumatology DH Unit; Chair, Department of Rheumatology, Gaetano Pini Institute, University of Milan, Italy

MASSIMO VARENNA, MD, PhD, Research Doctor, Rheumatology DH Unit; Chair, Department of Rheumatology, Gaetano Pini Institute, University of Milan, Italy

CONTENTS

Osteoporosis represents a major public health problem through its association with fragility fractures. Epidemiologic studies from North America estimated the remaining lifetime risk for common fragility fractures to be 17.5% for hip fracture, 15.6% for clinically diagnosed vertebral fracture, and 16% for distal forearm fracture among white women aged 50 years. Corresponding risks among men are 6%, 5%, and 2.5%, respectively. All osteoporotic fractures are associated with significant morbidity, but hip and vertebral fractures also are associated with excess mortality. Demographic changes can be expected to cause the number of hip fractures occurring worldwide to increase from 1.66 million in 1990 to 6.26 million in 2050.

Osteoporosis and related fragility fractures represent one of the most common complications that occurs in patients who have rheumatic diseases, and contributes to a dramatic decrease in quality of life. Bone is affected negatively by the disease process and often by the therapy itself in different rheumatic conditions, notably rheumatoid arthritis (RA), and the relationship between osteoporosis and osteoarthritis is a matter of concern. The clinical relevance of osteoporosis in rheumatic diseases is underestimated. Recent data demonstrated that patients who had RA and took oral corticosteroids did not undergo bone densitometry routinely. This article focuses on the burden of osteoporosis and fragility fractures in different rheumatic conditions, and emphasizes the importance of this complication for which effective preventive measures are available.

Genetics and Osteoporosis 659
Omar M.E. Albagha and Stuart H. Ralston

Osteoporosis is a common disease characterized by reduced bone mass and increased risk for fracture. Genetic factors play an important role in regulating bone mass, bone turnover, and bone geometry and also contribute to the pathogenesis of fracture by mechanisms independent of effects on bone density. In this article, the authors review the techniques that have been used to identify genes that regulate susceptibility to osteoporosis and discuss the major candidate genes that have been implicated in the regulation of bone mass and susceptibility to osteoporotic fracture.

Recommendations for Measurement of Bone Mineral Density and Identifying Persons to be Treated for Osteoporosis 681
Marc C. Hochberg

Clinical practice guidelines exist for the diagnosis and treatment of osteoporosis in men and postmenopausal women. These guidelines present a uniform set of recommendations. Unfortunately, studies have shown a low rate of screening and treatment, particularly in high-risk groups, such as patients who have experienced a fracture. It is hoped that quality improvement projects, such as that currently being conducted by the American Medical Association in conjunction with numerous specialty societies, will lead to an improvement in physician practices in this area that will result in a reduction in morbidity and mortality from osteoporotic fractures.

Emerging Issues With Bisphosphonates 691
Ian R. Reid

Bisphosphonates are the most commonly used agents in the management of metabolic bone diseases. Despite their established therapeutic value, a number of points of uncertainty remain, particularly in connection with their optimal long-term use. It is likely that definitive clinical trial data will not become available to resolve these questions, so careful clinical observation and caution are needed in patients who require treatment over periods of more than 10 years.

Parathyroid Hormone Update 703
Kendal L. Hamann and Nancy E. Lane

Osteoporosis afflicts an estimated 10 million United States citizens, and approximately one in two women and one in four men who are older than the age of 50 will suffer from an osteoporosis-related fracture in their remaining lifetimes. US Food and Drug Administration (FDA)-approved therapies for the treatment and prevention of osteoporosis include calcium and vitamin D supplements and antiresorptive therapies. Recombinant human parathyroid hormone (rhPTH) and recombinant bioactive fragments of human parathyroid hormone (PTH) are emerging as a unique new class of treatment options for osteoporosis. This article briefly reviews the physiology and rationale for the use of PTH for the treatment of osteoporosis, and provides a more detailed update on the application of recent clinical trials of PTH to clinical practice.

One of the major challenges for rheumatologists in the successful management of patients who have osteoporosis is poor patient adherence to current therapies. Patients who are nonadherent to osteoporosis therapies have significant consequences of reduced bone mineral density response, reduced bone marker suppression, and increased risk for osteoporotic fracture compared with patients who are adherent. Although extending the dosing interval of oral bisphosphonates from daily to weekly has improved adherence, adherence with weekly bisphosphonates remains suboptimal. Barriers to adherence include patient health beliefs, inadequate patient education, and age. Potential solutions include patient and family education, improved dosing schedules, and improved communication between patients and doctors.

Glucocorticoids (GCs) constitute a therapeutic class largely used in clinical medicine for the curative or supportive treatment of various conditions involving the intervention of numerous medical specialties. Beyond their favorable therapeutic effects, GCs almost invariably provoke bone loss and a rapid increase in bone fragility, with its host of fractures. Men and postmenopausal women constitute a preferential target for the bone complications of GCs. Exposure to GCs yields a fracture risk exceeding the risk conferred by a low bone mineral density per se. Nowadays, bisphosphonate therapy should be proposed to every patient at risk for fragility fracture, along with calcium and vitamin D supplementation. Studies of other therapeutic modalities (eg, promotors of bone formation) are in progress.

The inflammatory process in rheumatoid arthritis elicits intense bone loss that is manifest as articular bone erosions, juxta-articular osteopenia, and systemic osteoporosis. Key molecular discoveries coupled with elegant animal studies have highlighted a pathogenic role of osteoclasts in bone destruction. The tumor necrosis factor (TNF) family of cytokines, especially TNF-α and receptor activator of nuclear factor-κB ligand (RANKL), are pivotal for recruiting and activating osteoclasts and inducing bone loss. Targeted anti-TNF therapy or RANKL antagonism prevents inflammation-induced bone loss, and the potent new bisphosphonates are an emerging therapeutic tool.

FORTHCOMING ISSUES

RECENT ISSUES

THE CLINICS ARE NOW AVAILABLE ONLINE!

Access your subscription at:
http://www.theclinics.com

RHEUMATIC
DISEASE CLINICS
OF NORTH AMERICA

Rheum Dis Clin N Am 32 (2006) xi–xii

Preface

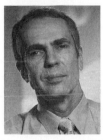

Philip N. Sambrook, MD
Guest Editor

This issue of the *Rheumatic Disease Clinics of North America* takes an in-depth look at key aspects of osteoporosis and presents significant advances that have occurred in the field recently. In particular, this issue gathers the work of a number of top researchers in the field to discuss epidemiology, clinical aspects of the disease, and treatment options, as well as emerging issues. There is a particular emphasis on glucocorticoid osteoporosis and the emerging field of osteoimmunology, which connects the fields of immunology and inflammatory bone loss.

The epidemiology of osteoporosis and the role of bone mineral density in the definition and prediction of fractures, as well as the most current information on the geographical distribution of the disease, are reviewed by Cyrus Cooper and Elaine Dennison. The issue also includes a thoughtful article by Luigi Sinigaglia devoted to the epidemiology of bone loss in inflammatory conditions such as rheumatoid arthritis, systemic lupus erythematosus, and ankylosing spondylitis. Genetic factors have been identified as playing an important role in the determination of bone mass and fractures, and recent advances in their role in osteoporosis are reviewed by Omar Albagha and Stuart Ralston.

Marc Hochberg reviews recommendations and algorithms for identifying persons who should undergo measurement of bone mass in an attempt to identify women and men with low mass who should undergo treatment to reduce their risk of fracture. Bisphosphonates are the most commonly used agents in the management of osteoporosis. Despite their established therapeutic value, a number of issues of uncertainty remain, particularly in

doi:10.1016/j.rdc.2006.11.001

connection with their optimal long-term use and toxicity. These emerging issues are discussed by Ian Reid. Anabolic agents, such as parathyroid hormone, and the use of combination and sequential therapies are also discussed in depth by Nancy Lane. Compliance with and adherence to osteoporosis therapies are increasingly recognized as issues in a disease process in which long-term therapy is required, and Stuart Silverman provides a thoughtful discussion on this topic.

For the rheumatologist, glucocorticoid osteoporosis is always an issue of concern, and Jean-Pierre Devogelaer provides an update on recent developments in this important topic. Finally, the pathogenesis and treatment of inflammation-induced bone loss are reviewed by Evange Romas.

Throughout this issue, there is an emphasis on advances in scientific knowledge as they relate to the biology of postmenopausal bone loss in women and inflammation-induced bone loss in both women and men, and on the diagnosis of and therapy for the prevention and treatment of osteoporosis.

Philip N. Sambrook, MD
University of Sydney
Institute of Bone and Joint Research
Level 4, Building 35 (Block 4)
Royal North Shore Hospital
St. Leonards, Sydney, Australia 2065

E-mail address: sambrook@med.usyd.edu.au

ELSEVIER
SAUNDERS

RHEUMATIC
DISEASE CLINICS
OF NORTH AMERICA

Rheum Dis Clin N Am 32 (2006) 617–629

Epidemiology of Osteoporosis

Elaine Dennison, MB, BChir, MA, MRCP, PhD*,
Maysam Abdin Mohamed, MB, BS, MRCP,
Cyrus Cooper, DM, FRCP, FMedSci

*MRC Epidemiology Resource Centre, Southampton General Hospital, Tremona Road,
Southampton SO16 6YD, United Kingdom*

Osteoporosis is a systemic skeletal disorder that is characterized by low bone mass and microarchitectural deterioration of bone tissue, with a consequent increase in bone fragility and susceptibility to fracture [1]. These fragility fractures have devastating health consequences through their association with increased mortality and morbidity, and consequently are a considerable burden to the health care system. Prospective studies indicate that the risk for osteoporotic fracture increases continuously as bone mineral density (BMD) declines, with a 1.5 fold to 3 fold increase in risk for fracture for each standard deviation decrease in BMD [2]. In the Rotterdam Study, a prospective, population-based cohort study of 7806 men and women aged 55 years or older, the age-adjusted hazard ratio per standard deviation decrease in femoral neck BMD was 1.5 for women and 1.4 for men [3]. Some risk factors for fragility fracture act through BMD (eg, female gender, Asian or white race, premature menopause, primary or secondary amenorrhea, primary and secondary hypogonadism in men, prolonged immobilization, low dietary calcium intake, and vitamin D deficiency) (Box 1). Several other factors contribute significantly to fracture risk over and above their association with BMD (high bone turnover, poor visual acuity, glucocorticoid therapy, family history of hip fracture). Fractures that are due to osteoporosis are found at areas that are typified by large amounts of trabecular bone; common fracture sites include the proximal femur (trochanteric fractures are associated more with osteoporosis than are cervical fractures), vertebrae, and distal radius. This article reviews the epidemiology of osteoporotic fracture.

---

* Corresponding author.
  E-mail address: emd@mrc.soton.ac.uk (E. Dennison).

0889-857X/06/$ - see front matter © 2006 Elsevier Inc. All rights reserved.
doi:10.1016/j.rdc.2006.08.003
rheumatic.theclinics.com

Box 1. Risk factors for fracture

Constitutional
Female gender
Age
Asian or white race
Sex hormone deficiency
Previous fragility fracture
Family history of fragility fracture
Early environment
Co-morbidity
Neuromuscular disorders

Lifestyle
Low body weight
Cigarette smoking
Excessive alcohol consumption
Prolonged immobilization
Low dietary calcium intake
Vitamin D deficiency

Absolute risks for fracture in individuals

Although most American women under the age of 50 years have normal BMD, 27% are osteopenic and 70% are osteoporotic at the hip, lumbar spine, or forearm by the age of 80 years. Epidemiologic studies from North America have estimated the remaining lifetime risk for common fragility fractures to be 17.5% for hip fracture, 15.6% for clinically diagnosed vertebral fracture, and 16% for distal forearm fracture among white women aged 50 years. Corresponding risks among men are 6%, 5%, and 2.5%, respectively. A recent British study, using the General Practice Research Database [4], estimated the lifetime risk for any fracture to be 53.2% at age 50 years among women, and 20.7% at the same age among men. Projected risks for fracture at various ages are displayed in Table 1. Site-specific lifetime risks at age 50 years are as follows: women—radius/ulna 16.6%, femur/hip 11.4%, and vertebral body 3.1%; men—radius/ulna 2.9%, femur/hip 3.1%, and vertebral body 1.2%. Among women, the 10-year risk for any fracture increased from 9.8% at age 50 years to 21.7% at age 80 years, whereas among men the 10-year risk remained stable with advancing age (7.1% at age 50 years and 8.0% at age 80 years). To put these figures in context, the estimated lifetime risk for endometrial carcinoma for a 50-year old woman is 2.6%, for breast cancer 10%, for coronary heart disease 46%, and for stroke 20% [5]. Our knowledge of the epidemiology of childhood fractures in the United Kingdom recently was expanded by interrogation of the same

Table 1
Estimated risks of fractures at various ages

	Current age (y)	Any fractures	Radius/ulna	Femur/hip	Vertebral
Lifetime risk					
Women	50	53.2%	16.6%	11.4%	3.1%
	60	45.5%	14.0%	11.6%	2.9%
	70	36.9%	10.4%	12.1%	2.6%
	80	28.6%	6.9%	12.3%	1.9%
Men	50	20.7%	2.9%	3.1%	1.2%
	60	14.7%	2.0%	3.1%	1.1%
	70	11.4%	1.4%	3.3%	1.0%
	80	9.6%	1.1%	3.7%	0.8%
10-Year risk					
Women	50	9.8%	3.2%	0.3%	0.3%
	60	13.3%	4.9%	1.1%	0.6%
	70	17.0%	5.6%	3.4%	1.3%
	80	21.7%	5.5%	8.7%	1.6%
Men	50	7.1%	1.1%	0.2%	0.3%
	60	5.7%	0.9%	0.4%	0.3%
	70	6.2%	0.9%	1.4%	0.5%
	80	8.0%	0.9%	2.9%	0.7%

Data from Van Staa TP, Dennison EM, Leufkens HGM, et al. Epidemiology of fractures in England and Wales. Bone 2001;29:520.

database; at their childhood peak, the prevalence of fractures (boys 3%, girls 1.5%) is surpassed only at 85 years of age among women and never among men (Fig. 1) [6].

Health impact of osteoporotic fracture

All osteoporotic fractures are associated with significant morbidity, but hip and vertebral fractures also are associated with excess mortality. A recent study estimated that there were 1.31 million new hip fractures in 1990, and the prevalence of hip fractures with disability was 4.48 million. There were 740,000 deaths estimated to be associated with hip fracture and 1.75 million disability-adjusted life-years lost, which represents 0.1% of the global burden of disease worldwide and 1.4% of the burden among women from the established market economies [7].

Mortality

For fractures of the femur/hip and vertebral body, previous studies showed clear evidence of excess mortality up to 5 years following fracture for both sexes, although fractures of the radius/ulna were associated with slight excess mortality among men only [8]. Although this may represent complications of the fracture and subsequent surgery for hip fractures, it is likely to reflect coexisting comorbidity in vertebral fracture sufferers. It has been estimated that 8% of men and 3% of women over 50 years of

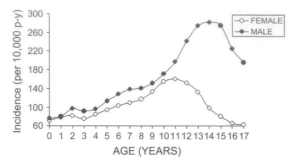

Fig. 1. Incidence of fractures among children from the General Practice Research Database. p-y, patient-year. (*From* Cooper C, Dennison EM, Leufkens HG, et al. Epidemiology of childhood fractures in Britain: a study using the General Practice Research Database. J Bone Miner Res 2004;19:1978; with permission of the American Society for Bone and Mineral Research.)

age die while hospitalized for their hip fracture; mortality continues to increase over the subsequent months, such that at 1 year, mortality is 36% for men (higher for the very elderly) and 21% for women [9]. By 2 years after hip fracture, mortality declines back to baseline, except in elderly patients and among men. The four main predictors for higher mortality seem to be male sex, increasing age, coexisting illness, and poor prefracture functional status.

Excess mortality after vertebral fracture seems to increase progressively after diagnosis of the fracture [10]. This has been observed in studies based on clinically diagnosed vertebral deformities and in those that used radiologic morphometric approaches to classify vertebral deformity. Impaired survival is more pronounced for vertebral fractures that follow moderate, rather than severe, trauma, of which only 8% is attributable to osteoporosis. Five-year survival seems to be worse for men (72%) than for women (84%). In women, an excess risk for death from cardiovascular and pulmonary disease that increases with increasing number of vertebral fractures has been observed [11].

Morbidity

A recent paper has weighted osteoporotic fracture according to their morbidity—loss in utilities—in relation to hip fractures, to obtain a definition of true burden of osteoporotic fracture [12]. Hence, to get the true morbidity expressed as the morbidity of hip fractures in men between the ages of 50 to 54 years, the incidence of hip fractures should be multiplied by 4.48. Thus, for men between 50 and 54 years, the disability that is caused by osteoporotic fractures is 4.48 times that accounted for by hip fracture alone. Four vertebral fractures have the same morbidity as does one hip fracture. For women of the same age, the incidence of hip fractures should be multiplied by a factor of 6.07. In the United States, about 7% of survivors of all types of fragility fractures have some degree of permanent disability, and

8% require long-term nursing home care. Overall, a 50-year-old white woman in the United States has a 13% chance of experiencing attributable functional decline after any fracture [13]. Hip fracture invariably requires hospitalization. The degree of functional recovery after this injury is age dependent; in the United States, 14% of patients in the 50- to 55-year age group who sustained a hip fracture were discharged to nursing homes, compared with 55% of those aged older than 90 years [13]. The length of stay also was related to age. Malnutrition, particularly of protein, may delay recovery significantly and is a common problem in the hospital environment. Premorbid status also is a strong predictor of outcome. In the United States, 25% of people who formerly were independent became at least partially dependent, 50% of those who were dependent before fracture were admitted to nursing homes, and those who already were in nursing homes remained there [14]. Results seem to be similar in France [15]. Hip fracture also has a significant effect on mobility; 1 year after hip fracture, 40% were unable to walk independently, 60% required assistance with at least one essential activity of daily living (eg, dressing, bathing), and 80% were unable to perform at least one instrumental activity of daily living (eg, driving, shopping) [9].

The impact of a single vertebral fracture may be low; however, multiple fractures cause progressive loss of height and kyphosis and severe back pain in the acute stages. The resultant loss of mobility can exacerbate underlying osteoporosis, which leads to the increased risk for further fractures [16]. The psychologic impact of functional loss can cause depression and social isolation as well as loss of self-esteem. Participants in the European Prospective Osteoporosis Study who had radiologically identified vertebral fracture at baseline and who suffered a further fracture during follow-up experienced substantial levels of disability with impairment in key physical functions of independent living [17].

Although good functional recovery after distal forearm fracture may be poor, reflecting complications (eg, reflex sympathetic dystrophy, neuropathies, posttraumatic arthritis), mortality after Colles' fracture does not deviate from the expected rate.

Economic cost

In the United Kingdom, the annual cost to the health care system from osteoporotic fracture has been estimated at 1.7 billion pounds, a significant contribution to the costs for Europe as a whole (13.9 billion Euros), and substantially lower than those for the United States (17.9 billion dollars). Hip fractures account for more than one third of the total figure, and reflect the cost of inpatient medical services and nursing home care. Expenditures are increasing faster than is the general rate of inflation, and they are a major source of concern to governmental leaders. Much research is focusing on the cost-effectiveness of treatment programs for osteoporosis; this remains difficult to assess, and in addition, the widespread use of expensive drugs may not be affordable in many countries. The cost of fracture is illustrated in Table 2.

Fracture epidemiology

Fracture incidence in the community is bimodal, with a peak in the young and elderly. In youth, fractures usually are associated with substantial trauma, occur in the long bones, and are seen more frequently in boys than in girls. Osteoporotic fractures characteristically occur in those areas of the skeleton with high amounts of trabecular bone after low or moderate trauma. There is increased frequency of fracture with age in both sexes, which reflects a combination of lower bone density with an increased tendency to fall in the elderly. Racial variation exists, with lower fracture rates observed in black populations than in white or Asian populations, although geographic variations in fracture rates have been demonstrated even within countries, which suggests that environmental factors also are important in the pathogenesis of hip fracture. A recent paper, using the US Study of Osteoporotic Fractures, examined the relationship between BMD and incident nonspinal fractures in 636 black and 7334 white women [18]. The absolute incidence of fracture across the pooled BMD distribution was 30% to 40% lower among black women at every BMD tertile. The lower risk for fracture among black women was independent of BMD and other lifestyle risk factors. The investigators speculated that it might be accounted for by slower rates of bone loss in black women, microarchitectural and geometric differences between ethnic groups, or differences in sex steroids or growth hormone levels.

The hip, spine, and distal forearm are the three sites that are associated most closely with osteoporotic fracture. The epidemiologic characteristics vary with each site as is discussed below.

Hip fracture

Several studies have suggested a wide geographic variation in hip fractures between, as well as within, countries. In general, people who live in latitudes further from the equator seem to have a higher incidence of fracture

Table 2
Costs associated with osteoporotic fracture

Site	Cost (US $)
Hip (first year)	21,000
Vertebral deformity	500
Clinical vertebral fracture	1200–3600

Data from Johnell O, Kanis J. Epidemiology of osteoporotic fractures. Osteoporos Int 2005;16:S3–7.

[19]. The highest rates of hip fracture are seen in white populations that live in northern Europe, especially Scandinavians, where the age-adjusted 1-year cumulative incidence in Norway in 1989 was 903/100,000 for women and 384/100,000 for men [20]. The rates are intermediate in Asians [21], in China [22], and in Kuwait [23], and are lowest in black populations [24]. Although studies in central Norway suggest stabilization in fracture rates in recent years [25], a Californian study reported a doubling of hip fracture rates in Hispanics, whereas no significant change occurred among black or Asian men or women [26]. Many of the lower incidence rates that are seen in developing countries can be explained, in part, by lower life expectancy; in Latin America, only 5.7% of the population is older than 65 years [27]. It was estimated that 1.66 million hip fractures occurred worldwide in 1990 [28], representing 1,197,000 fractures in women and 463,000 fractures in men. In Western populations, among individuals who are older than 50 years of age, there is a female preponderance of hip fracture, with a female/male incidence ratio of approximately 2:1.

Some interracial differences may be explained by variations in reversible lifestyle factors, such as low milk consumption, cigarette smoking, lack of sunlight exposure, low BMI, and physical activity; however, genetic factors also may be important. Various diseases that are associated with secondary osteoporosis and with falling seem to be a more important cause of hip fractures in men than in women.

Vertebral fracture

Until recently, accurate epidemiologic studies of vertebral fracture have been limited; this reflects the clinically silent nature of two thirds of these fractures, in addition to a lack of consensus regarding the techniques that should be used to define vertebral deformity [29]. The advent of descriptions of morphometric and semiquantitative visual techniques has enabled several studies to report the prevalence of vertebral fracture. Only about one third of all vertebral deformities that are noted on radiographs come to medical attention, and less than 10% necessitate admission to the hospital [30].

For example, in Rochester, Minnesota, the prevalence of any vertebral deformity was estimated at 25.3% per 100 women aged 50 years and older, whereas the incidence of a new deformity in this group was estimated at 17.8 per 1000 person-years [31]. By contrast, in the European Vertebral Osteoporosis Study, one in eight women and men aged 50 years and older had evidence of vertebral deformity [32]. The prevalence of vertebral deformity increased steadily with age in both sexes, although the gradient was steeper for women. There was a three-fold variation in the occurrence of deformity across Europe, and up to a two-fold variation in centers within individual countries; this may reflect a combination of environmental and genetic factors. The risk for vertebral deformity among men was elevated significantly in those with high levels of physical activity, which suggests the etiologic importance of trauma. By contrast, women with higher levels of customary physical activity had a reduced risk for deformity [33].

In instances in which comparable methods and definitions have been used in studies, the prevalence of vertebral fractures has been more similar across regions than that seen for hip fractures. For example, vertebral fracture prevalence among women in Hiroshima, Japan are 20% to 80% greater than for white women in Rochester, Minnesota, despite lower rates of hip fracture in the former group [34]. Similarly, the risk for vertebral fractures among postmenopausal women in Beijing, China is only 25% lower than that among women in Rochester, Minnesota, despite much lower rates of hip fracture in the former group [35]. Recent data from the Epidemiology of Osteoporosis Study yielded estimates of the prevalence of vertebral fractures to be 19% among women aged 75 to 79 years, 21.9% among women aged 80 to 84 years, and 41.4% among those aged 85 years and older; these are broadly in accord with estimates from other populations [36].

Only one quarter of vertebral fractures result from falls. Most are precipitated by routine daily activities (eg, bending or lifting light objects), which reflects the compressive load of such acts.

Wrist fracture

Distal forearm fracture usually results because of a fall onto an outstretched hand. These fractures show a steep increase in incidence during the perimenopausal period among women, but plateau thereafter. There is no apparent increase in the incidence of wrist fracture with age in men. In white women, the incidence increases linearly between the ages of 40 and 65 years, and then stabilizes; in men, the incidence remains constant between 20 and 80 years. A much stronger sex ratio exists for this fracture than for most others, and this has been estimated to be 4:1 in favor of women. Recent data from Dorset, United Kingdom showed that among women, the incidence of distal radius fracture increased from a premenopausal baseline of 10 per 10,000 population per year to a peak of 120 per 10,000 population per year over 85 years [37]. Although geographic variation exists, a partial explanation may be methodological considerations of case ascertainment, because less than 20% of patients who sustain forearm fractures are hospitalized. A winter peak is demonstrated again, but this probably is due to falls outside on icy surfaces. The plateau with age in women may be due to mode of falls; later in life, a woman is more likely to fall onto a hip than an outstretched hand because her neuromuscular coordination deteriorates.

Other fractures

The incidence of proximal humeral, pelvic, and proximal tibial fractures also increase steeply with age, and are greater in women than in men. Often, these are termed frailty fractures, because they typically occur in women who are losing weight involuntarily [38]. Furthermore, there is some direct evidence that these fractures are associated with low BMD [39]. Three quarters of all proximal humeral fractures are due to moderate trauma—typically a fall from standing height or less—and tend to be more common in women who have poor neuromuscular function [40].

Clustering of fractures

Previous vertebral deformities increase the risk for subsequent vertebral deformities by 7 to 10 fold (Table 3) [41,42]. This is similar to the increase in risk for a second hip fracture. In Rochester, Minnesota, residents aged 70 years or younger who had radiologically diagnosed vertebral deformities were followed for the development of subsequent limb fractures. The standardized morbidity ratios of observed/expected fractures for both sexes were 1.7 (95% CI, 1.3–2.2) for the hip, 1.4 (95% CI, 1.0–1.8) for the forearm, and 1.5 (95% CI, 1.3 1.8) for any limb fracture. This increased risk was more marked in subjects who had vertebral deformities that were associated with moderate or minimal trauma than with severe trauma [43].

The Study of Osteoporotic Fractures, a prospective study of 9704 United States women aged 65 years or older, also investigated the relationship between prevalent vertebral deformity and incident osteoporotic fracture [44]. Prevalent vertebral deformity (assessed morphometrically) was associated with a five-fold increased risk for sustaining a further vertebral deformity; the risk for hip fracture was increased 2.8-fold (95% CI, 2.3 3.4) and the risk for any nonvertebral fracture was increased 1.9-fold (95% CI, 1.7–2.1), after adjustment for age and calcaneal BMD. Although there was a small increased risk for wrist fracture, this was not significant after adjustment for age and BMD.

The Rochester Minnesota project also was used to ascertain the ability of distal forearm fractures to predict future fractures [45]. Among residents who experienced their first distal forearm fracture at age 35 years or older—and excluding fractures that occurred on the same day as the index forearm fracture—hip fracture risk was increased 1.4-fold in women (95% CI, 1.1–1.8) and 2.7-fold in men (95% CI, 0.98–5.8). Excess risk in women was confined to those individuals who sustained their first forearm fracture at age 70 years or older. By contrast, vertebral fracture was increased at all ages, with

Table 3
Number of prevalent vertebral deformities and risk for subsequent vertebral fracture

	No. of deformities		
	1	2	3 or more
Relative risk for subsequent vertebral fracture	3.2	9.8	23.3
95% CI	2.1–4.8	6.1–15.8	15.3–35.4

From Cooper C. Epidemiology of osteoporotic fracture: looking to the future. Rheumatology 2005;44:iv36–40; with permission.

a 5.2-fold (95% CI, 4.5–5.9) increase in risk among women and a 10.7-fold (95% CI, 6.7–16.3) increased risk among men.

Bone mineral density and fracture

The relationship between BMD and osteoporosis can be compared with that between blood pressure and stroke. Although low BMD is not a prerequisite for osteoporotic fracture, the risk for fracture is elevated considerably in the presence of low bone mass. Therefore, as with blood pressure, appropriate cut-off values can be defined to direct intervention toward "at-risk" individuals. BMD taken at different sites can be used to predict the future risk for fracture at the same, or other, sites.

Falls and fracture

Fractures occur because of an interaction between bone fragility (largely determined by bone mass) and trauma (usually falls). In particular, distal forearm fracture and hip fracture usually follow a fall from standing height or less. The likelihood of fall increases with age, especially for elderly women. In one British study based in Oxford, one in three women, aged 80 to 84 years, had experienced a fall in the previous year. Above this age, one half of the women and one third of the men had experienced a fall in the preceding year [46].

There are multiple factors that increase the likelihood of a fall, including use of medications, such as antidepressants and benzodiazepines [47,48], and coexistent illness. Physical activity may be protective. Only 1% of falls lead to a hip fracture, mainly because of the orientation of the fall. A fall sideways leads to direct impact on the greater trochanter and failure to break the fall with an outstretched hand [49].

Future projections

Osteoporotic fractures represent a significant public health burden, which is set to increase in future generations. Life expectancy is increasing worldwide, and it is estimated that the number of individuals aged 65 years and older will increase from the current figure of 323 million to 1555 million by the year 2050. These demographic changes alone can be expected to cause the number of hip fractures that occurs worldwide to increase from 1.66 million in 1990 to 6.26 million in 2050 [28]. Although one half of all hip fractures among elderly people in 1990 took place in Europe and North America, the rapid ageing of the Asian and Latin American populations suggests that 75% of hip fractures will occur there by 2050 [50]. In addition, although age-adjusted rates seem to have leveled off in the northern part of the United States and United Kingdom, rates continue to increase in countries, such as Hong Kong and Finland. Based on current trends, hip fracture rates might increase in the United Kingdom from 46,000 in 1985 to 117,000 in 2016.

Summary

Osteoporotic fractures represent a significant public health burden, which is set to increase in future generations. Lifetime risk is high and lies within the range of 40% to 50% in women and 13% to 22% in men. Life expectancy is increasing worldwide, and it is estimated that the number of individuals aged 65 years and older will increase from the current figure of 323 million to 1555 million by the year 2050. These demographic changes alone can be expected to cause the number of hip fractures occurring worldwide to increase from 1.66 million in 1990 to 6.26 million in 2050. Based on current trends, hip fracture rates might increase in the United Kingdom from 46,000 in 1985 to 117,000 in 2016. The societal cost of these fractures is high; cost-effectiveness analyses showed cost-effectiveness in treating high-risk patients with antiresorptive drugs, particularly if administered as soon as possible after a first fragility fracture.

References

[1] Consensus Development Conference. Prophylaxis and treatment of osteoporosis. Osteoporos Int 1991;1:114–7.

[2] World Health Organization. Assessment of fracture risk and its application to screening for postmenopausal osteoporosis. WHO Technical Report Series. Geneva (Switzerland): WHO; 1994.

[3] Schuit SC, van der Klift M, Weel AE, et al. Fracture incidence and association with bone mineral density in elderly men and women: the Rotterdam Study. Bone 2004;34:195–202.

[4] Van Staa TP, Dennison EM, Leufkens HGM, et al. Epidemiology of fractures in England and Wales. Bone 2001;29:517–22.

[5] Grady D, Rubin SM, Petitti DB, et al. Hormone therapy to prevent disease and prolong life in postmenopausal women. Ann Intern Med 1992;117:1016–37.

[6] Cooper C, Dennison EM, Leufkens HG, et al. Epidemiology of childhood fractures in Britain: a study using the General Practice Research Database. J Bone Miner Res 2004;19: 1976–81.

[7] Johnell O, Kanis JA. An estimate of the worldwide prevalence, mortality and disability associated with hip fracture. Osteoporos Int 2004;15:897–902.

[8] Cooper C, Atkinson EJ, Jacobsen SJ, et al. Population-based study of survival after osteoporotic fractures. Am J Epidemiol 1993;137:1001–5.

[9] Hip fracture outcomes in people aged fifty and over: mortality, service use, expenditures, and long-term functional impairment. Washington, DC: Office of Technology Assessment, Congress of the United States; 1993. US Dept of Commerce Publication NTIS PB94107653.

[10] Kado DM, Browner WS, Palermo L, et al. Vertebral fractures and mortality in older women: a prospective study. Arch Intern Med 1999;159:1215–20.

[11] Chrischilles EA, Butler CD, Davis CS, et al. A model of lifetime osteoporosis impact. Arch Intern Med 1991;151:2026–32.

[12] Kanis JA, Johnell O, Oden A, et al. The risk and burden of vertebral fractures in Sweden. Osteoporos Int 2004;15:20–6.

[13] Baudoin C, Fardellone P, Bean K, et al. Clinical outcomes and mortality after hip fracture: a 2-year follow-up study. Bone 1996;18(3 Suppl):149S–57S.

[14] Poor G, Atkinson EJ, O'Fallon WM, et al. Predictors of hip fractures in elderly men. J Bone Miner Res 1995;10:1900–7.

[15] Johnell O, Gullberg B, Kanis JA, et al. Risk factors for hip fracture in European women: The MEDOS Study. J Bone Miner Res 1995;10:1802–14.

[16] Gold DT. The clinical impact of vertebral fractures: quality of life in women with osteoporosis. Bone 1996;18(Suppl 3):S185–9.

[17] O'Neill TW, Cockerill W, Matthis C, et al. Back pain, disability, and radiographic vertebral fracture in European women: a prospective study. Osteoporos Int 2004;15:760–5.

[18] Cauley JA, Lui LY, Ensrud KE, et al. Bone mineral density and the risk of incident nonspinal fractures in black and white women. JAMA 2005;293:2102–8.

[19] Chang K, Center J, Nguyen TV, et al. Incidence of hip and other osteoporotic fractures in elderly men and women: Dubbo Osteoporosis Epidemiology Study. J Bone Miner Res 2004;19:532–6.

[20] Falch J, Aho H, Berglund K, et al. Hip fractures in Nordic cities: difference in incidence. Ann Chir Gynaecol 1995;84:286–90.

[21] Hagino H, Yamamoto K, Teshima R, et al. The incidence of fractures of the proximal femur and distal radius in Tottori Prefecture Japan. Arch Orthop Trauma Surg 1990;109:43–4.

[22] Yan L, Zhou B, Prentice A, et al. Epidemiological study of hip fracture in Shenyang Peoples Republic China. Bone 1999;24:151–5.

[23] Memon A, Pospula W, Tantawy A, et al. Incidence of hip fracture in Kuwait. Int J Epidemiol 1998;27:860–5.

[24] Solomon L. Osteoporosis and fracture of femoral neck in the South African Bantu. J Bone Joint Surg 1968;50:2–13.

[25] Finsen V, Johnsen LG, Trano G, et al. Hip fracture incidence in central Norway: a follow-up study. Clin Orthop 2004;419:173–8.

[26] Zingmond DS, Melton LJ III, Silverman SL. Increasing hip fracture incidence in California Hispanics, 1983 to 2000. Osteoporos Int 2004;15:603–10.

[27] Morales Torres J, Gutierrez-Urena S. The burden of osteoporosis in Latin America. Osteoporos Int 2004;15:625–32.

[28] Cooper C, Campion G, Melton LJ III. Hip fracture in the elderly: a world wide projection. Osteoporos Int 1992;2:285–9.

[29] Cooper C, Atkinson EJ, O'Fallon MW, et al. Incidence of clinically diagnosed vertebral fractures: a population-based study in Rochester, Minnesota, 1985–1989. J Bone Miner Res 1992;7:221–7.

[30] Cooper C, Melton LJ III. Vertebral fracture: how large is the silent epidemic? BMJ 1992;304:793–4.

[31] Melton LJ, Lane AW, Cooper C, et al. Prevalence and incidence of vertebral deformities. Osteoporos Int 1993;3:113–9.

[32] O'Neill TW, Felsenberg D, Varlow J, et al. The prevalence of vertebral deformity in European men and women: The European Vertebral Osteoporosis Study. J Bone Miner Res 1996;11:1010–7.

[33] Silman AJ, O'Neill TW, Cooper C, et al. Influence of physical activity on vertebral deformity in men and women: results from the European Vertebral Osteoporosis Study. J Bone Miner Res 1997;12:813–9.

[34] Ross PD, Fujiwara S, Huang C, et al. Vertebral fracture prevalence in women in Hiroshima compared to Caucasians or Japanese in the US. Int J Epidemiol 1995;24:1171–7.

[35] Ling X, Cummings SR, Mingwei Q, et al. Vertebral fractures in Beijing, China: the Beijing Osteoporosis Project. J Bone Miner Res 2000;15:2019–25.

[36] Grados F, Marcelli C, Dargent-Molina P, et al. Prevalence of vertebral fractures in French women older than 75 years from the EPIDOS study. Bone 2004;34:362–7.

[37] Thompson PW, Taylor J, Dawson A. The annual incidence and seasonal variation of fractures of the distal radius in men and women over 25 years in Dorset, UK. Injury 2004;35(5):462–6.

[38] Ensrud KE, Cauley J, Lipschutz R, et al. Weight change and fractures in older women. Arch Intern Med 1997;157:857–63.

[39] Seeley DG, Browner WS, Nevitt MC, et al. Which fractures are associated with low appendicular bone mass in elderly women? The Study of Osteoporotic Fractures Research Group. Ann Intern Med 1991;115:837–42.

[40] Kelsey JL, Browner WS, Seeley DG, et al. Risk factors for fractures of the distal forearm and proximal humerus. Am J Epidemiol 1992;135:477–89.

[41] Ross PD, Davis JW, Epstein R, et al. Pre-existing fractures and bone mass predict vertebral fracture incidence. Ann Intern Med 1991;114:919–23.

[42] Cooper C. Epidemiology of osteoporotic fracture: looking to the future. Rheumatology 2005;44:iv–iv40.

[43] Cooper C, Kotowicz M, Atkinson EJ, et al. Risk of limb fractures among men and women with vertebral fractures. In: Papapoulos SE, Lips P, Pols HAP, et al, editors. Osteoporosis. Amsterdam: Elsevier; 1996. p. 101–4.

[44] Black DM, Arden NK, Palermo L, et al. Prevalent vertebral deformities predict hip fractures and new vertebral deformities but not wrist fractures. J Bone Miner Res 1999;14:821–8.

[45] Cuddihy MT, Gabriel SE, Crowson CS, et al. Forearm fractures as predictors of subsequent osteoporotic fractures. Osteoporos Int 1999;9:469–75.

[46] Winner SJ, Morgan CA, Evans JG. Perimenopausal risk of falling and incidence of distal forearm fracture. BMJ 1989;298:2486–8.

[47] Liu B, Anderson G, Mittmann N, et al. Use of selective serotonin-reuptake inhibitors or tricyclic antidepressants and risk of hip fractures in elderly people. Lancet 1998;351:1303–7.

[48] Cumming RG. Epidemiology of medication-related falls and fractures in the elderly. Drugs Aging 1998;12:43–53.

[49] Parkkari J, Kannus P, Palvanen M, et al. Majority of hip fractures occur as a result of a fall and impact on the greater trochanter of the femur: a prospective controlled hip fracture study with 206 consecutive patients. Calcif Tissue Int 1999;65:183–7.

[50] Johnell O, Kanis J. Epidemiology of osteoporotic fractures. Osteoporos Int 2005;16:S3–7.

RHEUMATIC
DISEASE CLINICS
OF NORTH AMERICA

ELSEVIER
SAUNDERS

Rheum Dis Clin N Am 32 (2006) 631–658

Epidemiology of Osteoporosis in Rheumatic Diseases

Luigi Sinigaglia, MD[a],*, Massimo Varenna, MD, PhD[a],
Giuseppe Girasole, MD, PhD[b],
Gerolamo Bianchi, MD[b]

[a]Department of Rheumatology, Gaetano Pini Institute, University of Milan,
Via Gaetano Pini 7, 20122 Milan, Italy
[b]Bone Metabolic Unit, Department of Rheumatology, La Colletta Hospital,
Via del Giappone 3, 16011 Arenzano (Genova), Italy

Osteoporosis and related fragility fractures are one of the most common complications that occur in patients who have rheumatic diseases, and they contribute to a dramatic decrease in quality of life. Bone is affected negatively by the disease process and often by the therapy itself in different rheumatic conditions, notably rheumatoid arthritis (RA), but also systemic lupus erythematosus (SLE), ankylosing spondylitis (AS) and spondyloarthritides, various connective tissue diseases, and polymyalgia rheumatica, and the relationship between osteoporosis and osteoarthritis (OA) is a matter of concern. The clinical relevance of osteoporosis in rheumatic diseases is underestimated. Recent data demonstrated that patients who had RA and took oral corticosteroids did not undergo bone densitometry routinely (only 23% of 236 patients) and that only 42% were prescribed a medication to reduce bone loss (not including calcium and vitamin D) [1]. This reflects an insufficient appreciation of this clinical challenge by most physicians, and a general lack of consensus on appropriate screening and treatment for osteoporosis in rheumatic diseases. This article focuses on the burden of osteoporosis and fragility fractures in different rheumatic conditions, and emphasizes the importance of this complication for which effective preventive measures are available.

---

* Corresponding author.
E-mail address: sinigaglia@gpini.it (L. Sinigaglia).

0889-857X/06/$ - see front matter © 2006 Elsevier Inc. All rights reserved.
doi:10.1016/j.rdc.2006.07.002
rheumatic.theclinics.com

Rheumatoid arthritis

Epidemiology of osteoporosis in rheumatoid arthritis

Involvement of bone in RA was described first by Barwell in 1865 [2]. Since then it has been well known that generalized and iuxta-articular osteoporosis can occur in RA. The magnitude of generalized osteoporosis in RA is difficult to assess, and available data come from cross-sectional studies that aimed to evaluate the prevalence of this complication. When comparing different studies it is important to recognize potential problems in data interpretation that are related to inclusion criteria and the diverse methods and sites of bone density measurements. A large review that was published in 1996 was based on the analysis of 10 cross-sectional studies that included less than 100 patients each and were performed by different techniques including single- and dual-photon absorptiometry and quantitative CT (QCT). The only conclusion was that patients who had RA had lower bone mass in the appendicular and axial skeleton when compared with controls [3]. More recently, the results of larger cross-sectional studies that used dual-energy X-ray absorptiometry (DXA) became available. In a large cross-sectional study that was performed on 925 consecutive women who had RA (73% of whom were postmenopausal) and were recruited in 21 Italian rheumatology centers, the frequency of osteoporosis as assessed by DXA was as high as 28.8% at the lumbar spine and 36.2% at the femoral neck. It increased linearly from Steinbrocker's functional stage I to IV. Patients who had vertebral or femoral osteoporosis had a significantly lower body mass index, a significantly longer duration of disease, and a significantly higher grade of disability as compared with nonosteoporotic counterparts, even after adjusting for age [4]. Because these data reflect the prevalence of osteoporosis in a series of patients that were referred to rheumatologic units, it is possible that a selection bias led to an overestimation. In the attempt to overcome this problem, a large cross-sectional study was performed in Norway in 394 woman, aged 20 to 70 years, who were recruited from a validated RA register that contained mild and severe cases and was suggested to be representative of the total RA population in the country [5]. In this study, the prevalence of osteoporosis in the whole sample was lower (16.8% at lumbar spine and 14.7% at femoral neck) but it reached values as high as 31.5% and 28.6% for the lumbar spine and femoral neck, respectively, in older women (60–70 years). A twofold increased frequency of osteoporosis was observed in all age groups compared with the reference population.

Data on the prevalence of osteoporosis in men who have RA are scanty. A study that was performed on 50 consecutive men (median age, 67 years) who were affected by long-standing RA reported a prevalence of femoral and lumbar osteoporosis of 29% and 19%, respectively, and reduced bone mineral density (BMD) was independent of serum testosterone concentrations [6]. In another study that was performed on 104 men who had RA the overall prevalence was lower (10%–13%), but it increased to 42% when considering any site of measurement in the older group (aged 60–69 years) [7]. Another cross-sectional study that included 94 men who had RA explored the overall frequency of reduced BMD (defined as a Z score of ≤ 1 standard deviation below the mean value in controls). It reported a twofold, statistically significant increased frequency of patients with reduced bone mass in the spine and the hip. In this study, multivariate analysis did not reveal consistent associations between reduced BMD and demographic or disease-related variables [8].

As for primary osteoporosis, BMD in patients who have RA is influenced by several factors. Cross-sectional studies provide important information about the influence of time-invariant factors as determinants of osteoporosis in RA. The main studies that were conducted in this field by multivariate analysis are in substantial agreement. They indicate that age, body weight or body mass index, physical disability as measured by Health Assessment Questionnaire, and menopausal status are the most important statistically significant, independent predictors of BMD or osteoporosis at the lumbar spine or proximal femur in women who have RA [4,5]. Conversely, physical activity, as assessed by the Framingham activity index, correlated significantly with BMD in patients who had RA, it was found by multiple regression analysis to be a significant independent predictor of femoral bone density in 111 women [9]. These results were confirmed recently by a study that assessed the relationship between bone density and muscular function. After adjustment for confounding covariates, women who had RA and subnormal BMD of the femoral neck (eg, T-score < -1) had a 20% lower quadriceps strength than did those with normal BMD [10]. In agreement with other studies that indicated a relationship between BMD and surrogate measures of physical performance [11–14], these data underscore the importance of muscle strengthening programs in the prevention of bone loss in patients who have RA.

An even more intriguing question that is addressed by most cross-sectional studies relates to the role of therapies as determinants of BMD and osteoporosis in patients who have RA. In this respect, the interpretation of studies of patients who take low-dose oral corticosteroids is difficult because of the number of factors that can influence BMD in these patients. In general, patients who are on steroids are likely to have more severe disease and to be more disabled. Two cross-sectional studies that were performed by dual-photon absorptiometry failed to demonstrate a statistically significant difference in spinal or femoral BMD between women who had RA and took corticosteroids and those who did not. It was concluded that low-dose prednisolone (mean daily dose of 6.6–8.5 mg) was not associated with an increased risk for osteoporosis [15,16]. Subsequent studies that used QCT or DXA gave controversial results. In a cross-sectional study of 74 patients who had RA, patients who were on oral corticosteroids had a 31% and 37% reduction in spinal trabecular and cortical BMD, respectively, compared with patients who did not undergo steroid treatment [17]. A DXA study that was performed on 195 postmenopausal patients who had RA showed that current steroid usage led to a significant reduction in BMD, and that groups that took low and high cumulative doses were at risk for decreased BMD as compared with ex-users or nonusers [18]. Conversely, a recent cross-sectional study performed by DXA on 146 women who had RA came to the conclusion that long disease duration, severity of disease, and decreased lean body mass, but not corticosteroids, were associated with generalized osteoporosis [19]. These results were confirmed by others that used skeletal ultrasonography [20]. In another study that was performed on 120 postmenopausal elderly women, current users of steroids had the lowest BMD at the distal forearm, calcaneus, and hip; however, functional outcomes of RA mostly accounted for these results [21]. Conversely, the two largest cross-sectional studies that were performed in the last years agree that current use of steroids is an independent predictor of reduced lumbar and femoral BMD [5] and osteoporosis [4], and that a low-dose steroid regimen (current dose of 5.5 ± 4.5 mg in prednisone equivalent) is associated with a 50% increase in the risk for osteoporosis [4]. In the Norwegian cohort study that was published by Haugeberg and colleagues [5] the prevalence of osteoporosis at lumbar spine raised from 8.6% in never users to 10.1% in previous and to 26.6% in current steroid users. These results are in agreement with data from a recent meta-analysis on the skeletal effect of corticosteroids that found strong correlations between cumulative doses of oral steroids and loss of BMD and between daily dose and the risk for fracture independent of underlying disease, age, and gender. This led to the conclusion that oral corticosteroid treatment of more than 5 mg of prednisone daily is able to reduce BMD with a rapid increase in the risk for fracture during the treatment period [22]. Finally, it was demonstrated recently in a randomized, placebo-controlled trial in healthy postmenopausal females that prednisone, 5 mg/d, rapidly and significantly suppressed multiple indices of bone formation. This suggests that even low doses may have adverse effects on bone mass or bone strength [23]. Table 1 summarizes the main results of the largest cross-sectional studies on the role of corticosteroids on bone mass in RA.

Besides low-dose corticosteroids, other agents that are used commonly in RA (eg, methotrexate) have been reported to exert a detrimental effect on the skeleton. In a recent large cross-sectional study that was performed on 533 postmenopausal women who had RA, however, the logistic regression model did not show any significant association between methotrexate use and the risk for osteoporosis [24].

Longitudinal surveys on osteoporosis in RA provide information about time-variant factors that influence bone mass. The first message from these prospective studies is that patients of both sexes who have RA effectively

Table 1
The effect of low-dose corticosteroids on bone mineral density in rheumatoid arthritis: results
from the main cross-sectional studies performed by dual-energy x-ray absorptiometry technique

Reference	N	Menopausal status	Current use of CS (%)	Role of CS
Hall et al, 1993 [18]	195 (F)	All Pm	21	Cumulative CS dose was a significant determinant of reduced BMD at the hip
Lane et al, 1995 [21]	120 (F)	All Pm	17.5	Lower appendicular and axial bone mass in current users
Haugeberg et al, 2000 [5]	394 (F)	66% Pm	40.5	Current use of CS was a predictor of BMD at FN and LS
Haugeberg et al, 2000 [8]	94 (M)		49.5	Current use of CS nonsignificant
Sinigaglia et al, 2000 [4]	925 (F)	73.3% Pm	68.2	Use of CS significantly associated with the risk for osteoporosis
Sambrook et al, 2001 [20]	76 (67F/9M)	Not reported	52.6	CS use was associated with small but nonsignificant reduction in BMD
Shibuya et al, 2002 [19]	146 (F)	All Pm	33.6	CS administration had no effect on BMD
Tengstrand & Hafstrom 2002 [7]	104 (M)		36	No correlation between BMD and CS treatment
Lodder et al, 2004 [32]	373 (288F/85M)	63.5% Pm	79	Use of CS was not associated independently with BMD

Abbreviations: CS, corticosteroids; F, female; FN, femoral neck; LS, lumbar spine; M, male
Pm, postmenopausal.

lose bone. In a population-based cohort of 366 patients who had RA and received conventional health care, the mean reduction in BMD over 2 years ranged from 0.29% at the spine to 0.77% at the total hip. In this study, treatment variables had a crucial role in the process of bone loss. Corticosteroid use was associated independently with an increased risk for BMD loss at the total hip (OR, 2.63) and at the lumbar spine (OR, 2.70), and the current use of antiresorptive drugs (including hormone replacement therapy, bisphosphonates, and calcitonin) were associated with a decreased risk for bone loss at the total hip (OR, 0.43) [25]. The second message strongly suggests that bone loss in RA is an early phenomenon. In one study of 67 subjects who had nonsteroid-treated RA of less than 5 years, patients with disease duration of less than 6 months had significantly greater loss of BMD at the femoral neck than did the remainder of the cohort over a 12-month period [26]. Finally, the most important message was the detrimental effect that uncontrolled disease activity had on bone density. A persistently elevated acute-phase response expressed by C-reactive protein levels was the single best predictor of BMD over 2 years in 148 patients who had early RA [27]; suppression of disease activity stabilized the bone loss. Differences in disease activity could explain the apparent lack of any detrimental effect of corticosteroids on bone in this series of patients who had early RA, in which the adverse effect on bone may be outweighed by an improved disease control by these hormones. From this perspective, suppression of disease activity probably remains the main concern when considering treatment options for osteoporosis in RA. This issue has been addressed by a few studies that showed that early treatment with disease-modifying drugs (DMARDs) has a significant sparing effect on metacarpal osteoporosis in RA [28], and that control of disease activity—in a group of patients that had active RA and started on DMARDs—can limit disease-associated bone loss as assessed by DXA [29]. Recently, over 54 weeks, aggressive treatment with a tumor necrosis factor α–blocking agent in RA of less than 12 months' duration exerted a protective effect against bone loss at the hip in a small group of patients [30].

Several studies have underscored the association between low bone mass and radiographic damage, which suggests a common mechanism for local and generalized osteoporosis in RA [31]. In the authors' [4] study that was performed on 925 women who had RA, the presence of erosions was associated with a significantly higher prevalence of osteoporosis at the lumbar or femoral level. Subsequent cross-sectional studies confirmed these results, which indicates that the presence of erosions and high Larsen scores for hands and feet is associated significantly with low BMD in both sexes [7,32,33]. Similar results were reported in a recent prospective study that demonstrated that BMD was correlated significantly with Larsen scores at baseline and after 2 years of disease in 134 women who had early RA [34]. This supports the assumption of a central role of osteoclastic activation as a common pathophysiologic mechanism that leads to secondary osteoporosis in RA [35]. To strengthen this link, it was reported recently that an increased urinary level of CTX-I, a marker of degradation of type I collagen in bone, was an important predictor of new joint damage over a 4-year follow-up period (relative risk of 15) in patients who had very early RA, in whom no joint damage could be detected radiographically at baseline [36]. Finally, in a multicenter study that was performed in three geographically close European countries on 150 women who had long-standing RA, multiple regression analysis showed that Larsen score was the independent determinant of vertebral deformities after correction for center, age, body mass index, and BMD [37].

Fractures in rheumatoid arthritis

Several reports indicated that fracture risk is increased in patients who have RA. The first population-based study that directly estimated fracture risk among patients who had RA was published 20 years ago. It reported relative risk (RR) estimates that achieved statistical significance only for pelvic fractures (RR, 2.56) and proximal femur fractures (RR, 1.51) [38]. In this study, no relative risk for vertebral fractures could be calculated because of the absence of incidence rates that allowed the determination of the expected number of fractures. Ten years later, the morphometric profile of spine radiographs in 76 postmenopausal women who had steroid-treated RA was compared with a sample of age-matched women from a population-based group. Vertebral fracture risk was increased considerably in RA, particularly in women aged 50 to 59 years, with an OR for the whole population that was as high as 6.2 [39]. A recent study definitely demonstrated that patients who have RA have more vertebral deformities than do population-based controls, with a high significant difference between patients and controls when multiple (OR 2.60) and moderate or severe deformities (OR 2.00) were considered [40]. In a population-based case-control study that was performed on 300 consecutive patients who had hip fracture compared with age- and sex-matched community controls, the crude risk for hip fracture was approximately doubled among patients who had RA; it increased markedly with increasing functional impairment [41]. More recently, a study that was performed in Finland reported an age- and sex-adjusted risk for hip fracture of 3.26 in 29 patients who had RA [42]. Recently, an OR of 9.0 for self-reported hip fracture was found in a cross-sectional case-control study that included 249 patients who had RA [43].

Factors that are associated with fractures in RA have been the subject of several studies. In a prospective study of 1110 patients of both genders who had RA and were followed for 8.4 years, variables that were associated with fracturing included years of taking prednisone, previous diagnosis of osteoporosis, a high disability index, older age, and little physical activity [44]. With respect to vertebral fractures, data from recent cross-sectional studies indicate that the presence of vertebral deformity was associated independently with age, longer than 12-month corticosteroid use, history of nonvertebral fracture, and low bone mass at total hip [45]. Finally, a 1-point increase in HAQ score was associated with a 70% increase in the risk for vertebral fracture in 461 cases of RA [4].

Few studies addressed the issue of falls and tendency to fall in RA. In a cross-sectional study in which fall risk factors were used as surrogates, fall-related risk factors that were predictive for hip fracture were three times more prevalent in patients who had RA as compared with the controls. Level of disability and tender joint count were the factors that had the most significant association with fall risk [46]. In another study that focused on fear of falling among patients who had RA, predictors for fear of falling and the major correlates for falls included greater pain intensity, lower functional status, and the number of comorbid conditions that accompanied RA [47].

The final question relates to the cost-effectiveness of identifying patients who have RA and are at risk for osteoporosis and fractures. Data have been published in an attempt to create a clinical algorithm to select postmenopausal women who have RA for bone densitometry in the aim to establish a treatment threshold. A five-item criteria set that is based on age (>50 years), weight (<60 kg), inflammation (as assessed by erythrocyte sedimentation rate and C-reactive protein levels), immobility (defined as HAQ≥ 1.25), and ever use of corticosteroids was tested in a cohort of patients that was believed to be representative of the entire RA population. It provided a practical tool to identify patients who had RA who should have a DXA measurement performed, with a sensitivity of 83% and a specificity of 45% [48].

Systemic lupus erythematosus

Epidemiology of osteoporosis in systemic lupus erythematosus

The outstanding improvement in the survival rates of patients who have SLE that has been achieved over the last few decades has directed attention to the morbidity that is associated with the disease and its treatment in long-term survivors. Many researchers have focused their attention on bone loss in these patients, and an increasing number of studies has been published recently on osteoporosis in patients who have SLE.

Pathogenetically, SLE could result in bone loss through several mechanisms that, in part, depend on the disease itself, and, in part, are treatment related (Box 1). Disease-dependent mechanisms include reduced physical activity secondary to long-standing disabling arthritis or myopathy, renal

---

Box 1. Potential mechanisms of bone loss in systemic lupus erythematosus

Disease dependent
Reduced motility
Renal impairment
Endocrine factors
Amenorrhea
Premature menopause
Low plasma androgen levels
Hyperprolactinemia
Chronic induction of bone-resorbing cytokines

Treatment dependent
Long-term corticosteroids
Immunosuppressive drugs
Azathioprine
Cyclophosphamide
Cyclosporin
Chronic anticoagulation
Avoiding sunshine

failure, endocrine dysfunctions, and the systemic effect of proinflammatory bone-resorbing cytokines. Besides corticosteroids, which are the mainstay of treatment in SLE, several other medications, such as azathioprine, cyclophosphamide, cyclosporin, and the long-term use of anticoagulants, can contribute to bone loss in these patients. Finally, counseling to avoid sunshine exposure can induce vitamin D deficiency, and, thus, contribute to reduced bone mass [49].

As for RA, studies on bone mass in SLE have some limitations and are difficult to compare in that they have different research designs, used different techniques and sites for measuring BMD, and included small numbers of patients of both sexes, women in the pre- or postmenopausal state and patients who had always or never been treated with corticosteroids. Most of the studies that have been published in the recent literature are of cross-sectional design, and share some further limitations because these observational models do not allow for the evaluation of risk factors for low bone mass, such as disease activity, which may change over time. Conversely, the few longitudinal studies that were performed on patients who had long-standing disease may have missed the effect of chronicity and treatment on the individual's bone density. The main controversies among the above mentioned cross-sectional studies are related to the prevalence of osteoporosis in patients who have SLE; the dependence or independence of this complication on glucocorticoid use is under debate as well. With the exception of the first study that was performed with DXA, in which lumbar BMD values in a small sample of premenopausal women who had SLE was found to be comparable with controls [50], all subsequent studies that were performed by the DXA technique found the mean BMD values in premenopausal women who had SLE to be significantly lower than in controls at the lumbar spine and at the proximal femur. In a study that was performed on 47 premenopausal women who had SLE, the most important finding was that patients who had never been treated with glucocorticoids had a lower hip BMD as compared with controls, which indicates that the disease, *per se*, may induce bone loss [51]. These data are consistent with a separate analysis of patients who had SLE who had not been treated with steroids that was reported in 1996 [52]. A modest loss of BMD was seen at the spine, hip, and forearm, which suggests that osteopenia in patients who have SLE may be disease related. Four studies failed to find any dependency of low bone mass in patients who had SLE and were taking corticosteroids [53–56]. This conclusion was reached by comparing BMD values between patients who had or who had never been treated with corticosteroids, or by searching for correlations between cumulative or current doses of prednisone and BMD. The comparison between patients who had or had not been treated with steroids must be regarded with caution, however, because patients who do not require steroids are likely to have milder forms of SLE. This point was addressed recently in a large cross-sectional study that was performed on 307 women who had SLE [57]. By multiple linear regression analysis, the investigators found significantly reduced BMD at the hip and lumbar spine in patients who had disease damage assessed by the SLICC score and who had ever received corticosteroids compared with women who did not have disease damage, but similar in amount to those who had damage and no corticosteroid exposure. Even if the group of corticosteroid-naive patients who had disease damage was small, because it is clinically uncommon, these results may support the hypothesis that there is an inverse association between disease damage and BMD in women who have SLE that is independent of corticosteroid use.

Conversely, most cross-sectional studies that focused on steroid treatment in SLE found that corticosteroids are the major determinants of low bone mass in patients who have SLE. Pons and coworkers [58] found that lumbar and femoral BMD were significantly lower in patients who were treated with prednisone dosages of at least 7.5 mg/d, with an overall prevalence of osteoporosis as high as 18% in steroid users. Another study in 97 premenopausal women who had SLE emphasized the role of corticosteroid exposure [59]. The investigators reported that cumulative steroid dose, the duration of steroid treatment, and the peak and current steroid dosage were associated significantly with low lumbar or femoral BMD, even after controlling for disease-related variables. The prevalence of osteoporosis in this study was 13.4% at the lumbar spine and 6.3% at the hip. An Italian study that was performed on 84 premenopausal women who had SLE found an overall prevalence of osteoporosis as high as 22.6%, and demonstrated that patients who had SLE and osteoporosis had a longer disease duration, higher cumulative steroid intake, longer steroid exposure, and higher disease severity as assessed by the SLICC/ACR score [60]. In the stepwise logistic regression analysis, 1 year of prednisone increased the risk for osteoporosis by 16%. In another cross-sectional study that was performed on 242 premenopausal women who had SLE, 10.3% of patients were in the osteoporotic range and exposure to prednisolone of more than 10 mg daily was associated significantly with reduced BMD [61]. In this study, Afro-Caribbean race was protective against reduced BMD—in agreement with other reports of a much lower prevalence of osteoporosis in non-Caucasian populations that have SLE [55,62]—which may be related to interethnic differences. Furthermore, patients who have childhood-onset SLE have a higher frequency of osteopenia as compared with age- and sex-matched controls. Also, the cumulative dose of corticosteroids was an important explanatory variable for bone mineral content in the lumbar spine and femoral neck of this particular group of patients [63]. Finally, the most extensive report of osteoporosis in patients who had SLE was published by Petri [64] in 1995 as part of an update analysis on musculoskeletal complications in the Hopkins Lupus Cohort. The sample included 407 patients, but no data were reported on the sex distribution and menopausal status. This study found a strong association of BMD at the lumbar spine with the cumulative and the highest prednisone dose. In the multiple regression model, patients who had SLE who were older, female, Caucasian, weighed less, had lower serum C4 levels, and who had taken prednisone in higher doses had lower BMD in the lumbar spine. Prednisone use remained an independent predictor of lumbar BMD, even after adjusting for all of the significant covariates.

Taken together, data from cross-sectional studies underscore the variable prevalence of osteoporosis in premenopausal women who have SLE, and its link with disease severity and corticosteroid treatment. A selection bias in DXA referral could account, at least in part, for prevalence data variability among different cross-sectional studies. In a sample of 516 women who had SLE, the group of patients that was referred for DXA scans were, on average, older, had increased lupus disease activity, and used more immunosuppressants [56]. In the only study that was performed on postmenopausal women who had SLE, the prevalence of osteoporosis at the lumbar spine was as high as 48% [65].

Few studies on bone mass in SLE have reported longitudinal results. Formiga and coworkers [66] repeated the measurements of bone mass in 25 consecutive patients, all of whom had continued on corticosteroid treatment. After 18 months there was no significant decrease in BMD at the lumbar spine or the femoral neck. Similar results were reported by another study in 21 patients who had SLE after 2-years of follow-up [67]. In another follow-up study on 32 women who had SLE, a daily dosage of prednisone of at least 7.5 mg was associated with a yearly loss of lumbar spine BMD not exceeding 0.5% [68]. A small, but significant, loss in the lumbar spine was detected after 1 year of observation in 20 younger patients who were affected with juvenile SLE and treated with steroids [69]. In summary, these studies, which were performed on small groups of patients in different stages of disease, indicate that the sequential loss of lumbar spine and femoral neck BMD in premenopausal women who have SLE is minimal. As has been reported in RA [26], however, rapid bone loss may occur at the onset of the disease, and, therefore, only can be detected in an inception cohort. A study that was performed on a small sample of premenopausal women who had a short disease duration of SLE showed a significant reduction of BMD at the lumbar spine and at Ward's triangle compared with age-matched healthy controls [70].

Osteoporosis in men who have SLE has received much less attention than in women. This issue was addressed specifically in a study that was performed on 20 patients and controls; no significant decrease in BMD was detected at the lumbar spine or at the femoral neck. The investigators did not find any correlation between androgen levels and BMD in this series; on the basis of this preliminary study they concluded that there is no evidence of bone loss in male patients who have SLE and are on corticosteroid therapy [71].

Fractures in systemic lupus erythematosus

Data on fractures in SLE are scanty. In the report that was published by Petri [64], the total number of fractures was 32 in 364 patients; 24 of these were defined as atraumatic. Predictors of fractures included age at the time of the study, the cumulative and highest dose of prednisone, avascular necrosis of bone, postmenopausal status, and the previous identification of osteopenia on any radiograph. Vertebral deformities that were scored with a semiquantitative method were detected in 20% of 107 pre- and postmenopausal women who had SLE [72] and in 21.4% of 70 premenopausal patients [73]. The most extensive retrospective, population-based study on self-reported fractures in 702 women who had lupus and were followed for 5951 person-years stated that the fracture risk was increased in the cohort that had lupus, as compared with control women of similar age, with a standardized morbidity ratio of 4.7 (95% CI, 3.8–5.8) [74]. Variables that were associated significantly with fracture were older age at diagnosis, longer disease duration, longer corticosteroid exposure, less use of oral contraceptives, and menopause. In the multivariate model only older age at lupus diagnosis and a longer duration of corticosteroid use were independent determinants of fractures. Furthermore, almost 50% of fractures occurred in women who had lupus who were younger than 50 years or premenopausal.

In conclusion, the high prevalence of osteoporosis that is reported by most studies and the impressive increase in the fracture rate in patients who have SLE represents an important challenge for clinicians. Strategies to counteract bone loss in SLE must be applied soon after disease onset, and include effective treatment of the underlying disease, modification of any known risk factor for osteoporosis, use of corticosteroids at the lowest useful dosage, and the pharmacologic treatment of osteoporosis in all patients with evidence of rapid bone loss.

Epidemiology of osteoporosis and fractures in ankylosing spondylitis

AS is the prototypical disease of a heterogeneous group of rheumatic disorders, which is called spondyloarthropathies (SspAs), that shares chronic inflammation of the axial skeleton as a common feature. Despite extraosseous new bone formation being considered a hallmark of AS, osteoporosis is a well-recognized feature that occurs even in the early, mild form of AS and leads to an increased rate of fractures. Radiographic bone loss has long been recognized in predensitometric studies [75,76], in which osteoporosis correlated with disease duration and older age. Studies that used direct assessment of BMD by means of different bone densitometry techniques have been reported extensively in the last decades. They yield inconsistent results about the real prevalence of osteoporosis in patients who have AS, probably because of the different tools that were used for evaluating bone mass, the cut-off chosen to define osteoporosis, and some variables that are related to the disease itself (eg, mean age of patients, the disease duration, anatomic evolution of AS).

Taken together, all studies that were performed by DXA at the lumbar level reported a decreased bone mass in early AS, in patients who had normal spine mobility and normal or increased levels of exercise, before the radiologic appearance of syndesmophytes, interapophyseal joint ankylosis, and ligamentous ossification [77,78]. In the same way, patients who had clinically mild disease without radiographic anatomic evolution showed a reduced BMD, despite having a longer disease duration [79]. These results suggest that bone loss occurs rapidly in AS, involves trabecular bone [80], and is not the simple consequence of spinal stiffness or immobility. Nevertheless, most studies demonstrated that even a cortical site (eg, femoral neck) showed a reduced BMD with decreases that seem to be related inversely to disease severity and duration [78], even if femoral neck BMD reduction seems to be more difficult to assess in early disease [80] and a possible hip involvement in AS represents a variable that is not evaluated in many studies. Femoral neck BMD in men was reported to be approximately 10% lower than in controls [77,81], with Z scores of around -1.073 [79]. Conversely, there is a general agreement that in advanced AS, lumbar BMD as measured by DXA, seems to be normal or even increased in comparison with the BMD of patients who have early AS and healthy controls [82,83]. This misleading increase and the discrepancy between lumbar and femoral neck BMD is due to the anatomic progression of AS; new bone formation increases the peripheral layer of vertebral bone, which masks the trabecular bone loss.

For these reasons, although lumbar DXA is the best tool to identify and to monitor patients who have early or mild disease, alternative techniques have been proposed in later stages of disease. QCT allows a selective measurement of vertebral trabecular bone, and showed a striking reduction of bone mass in patients who had severe AS who did not have decreased lumbar BMD values as assessed by DXA [80,84,85]. Differently from DXA, QCT shows a continued steady bone loss along with the anatomic disease progression [85,86]; however, the high costs and high radiation dose are regarded as disadvantages. The latest generation of DXA scanners incorporates supine lumbar lateral scanning software. This technique has the advantage of isolating the body of the L3 vertebra from anterior and posterior syndesmophytes and the ankylosed posterior elements of the spine. Although this tool also is more sensitive in detecting bone loss in long-standing AS [81,87] with a good correlation with femoral neck BMD, its value remains to be determined because of the lack of normative data, the higher precision error, and some technical difficulties that can arise in severely kyphotic patients (superposition of ribs or iliac crest).

Besides women who were included in mixed study groups [78,84,88], two studies that investigated BMD in women [89,90] showed a lower reduction of bone mass, probably as a result of less active disease as observed frequently in the female sex. Finally, patients with spinal involvement associated with other SspAs often have been included as small subgroups in larger samples of patients who have AS. In general, these subjects showed no difference in comparison with patients who did not have associated bowel disease, psoriasis, and reactive arthritis, even if a study on bone markers seemed to demonstrate some differences in bone metabolism in patients who had SspAs [91].

Taken together, the results of these studies are consistent with a systemic process that is related to the disease itself that affects bone metabolism, not only by changes in mechanical stress that are related to spinal stiffness or immobility as proposed for advanced AS. The few longitudinal studies on BMD demonstrated a greater bone loss in patients who had active disease and a correlation between serum inflammatory parameters, bone resorption markers, and BMD decreases [92,93]. Because of all of these issues, it is not surprising that the literature offers inconsistent results about the association between osteoporosis and AS, with a prevalence ranging from 18.7% [94] to 62% [75].

As a consequence of osteoporosis, vertebral compression fractures are reported frequently in AS, even if in clinical practice they probably are underdiagnosed, because the pain associated with them is attributed to exacerbations of the spondylitic process. It seems likely that the wide range of reported prevalence of vertebral fractures is related to the different methods that are used to define vertebral fractures and differences in patient selection (Table 2). Also, some anatomic findings that are related to AS (spondilodyscitis or Romanus lesion) can give a spurious appearance of vertebral wedging. Despite the pathogenetic mechanisms of osteoporosis that

Table 2
Prevalence of vertebral fractures in ankylosing spondylitis

Reference	N	Mean age (y)	Sex ratio (male/female)	Disease duration (y)	Prevalence of vertebral fractures (%)
Hanson et al, 1971 [75]	50	Range: 29–75	40/10	NA	4
Donnelly et al, 1994 [78]	87	44	62/25	16	10.3
Mitra et al, 2000 [79]	66	44	66/0	9.8	16.7
Devogelaer et al, 1992 [84]	70	39 Men 35 Women	60/10	15.4 Men 13.1 Women	4.2
Toussirot et al, 2001 1994 [88]	71	39	49/22	10.6	1.4
Cooper et al, 1994 [95]	158	33.8	121/37	NA	9.5
Ralston et al, 1990 [96]	111	41	98/13	17	18
Sivri et al, 1996 [100]	22	36	20/2	9.8	40.9
Baek et al, 2005 [101]	76	28	76/0	9.4	3.9

Abbreviation: NA, not assessed.

seem to involve the entire skeleton through a systemic inflammatory process, an increased rate of appendicular osteoporotic fractures has never been reported, and vertebral fractures seem to be the only clinical consequence of osteoporosis in patients who have AS. The early increase in the vertebral fracture risk within 5 years of diagnosis of AS [95] is consistent with densitometric studies that demonstrated a significant bone loss in early disease. Nevertheless, neither lumbar nor femoral BMD is a good predictor of the likelihood of fracture [78,79]. This issue probably is related to the reported bias in lumbar DXA measurement in advanced stages and a lack of site specificity for femoral neck evaluation. The only study that was able to quantify the fracture risk in patients who had AS was published by Cooper and colleagues [95]. Through a retrospective population-based study, they showed an increased vertebral fracture risk as great as 7.6 (95% CI, 4.3–12.6) in comparison with the expected fracture incidence in the same community.

In general, vertebral fractures in AS occur with increasing age, disease duration, and severity of disease [78,79,95], and show the greatest prevalence 2 to 3 decades after diagnosis. It is likely that compression fractures contribute—independently of the severity of the disease—to spinal deformity and decreased mobility of the spine and chest. With respect to the site of vertebral fractures, midthoracic vertebrae and the thoracolumbar passage are affected most commonly [96].

In addition to compression fractures, transverse and transdiscal fractures may occur in patients who have advanced AS [97] that also involve the cervical spine [98], with a reported higher rate of neurologic complications [99]. Changes in the pattern of mechanical stresses within an ankylosed and rigid spine are considered to be responsible for this particular kind of vertebral fracture.

Systemic sclerosis

Systemic sclerosis (SSc) is a connective tissue disorder that is characterized by fibrosis, degenerative changes, and vascular lesions of the skin with internal organ involvement. Several studies reported that SSc is associated with osteoporosis by different possible pathogenetic mechanisms. Besides a chronic inflammation state, a reduced bone mass in patients who have SSc could be related to a decreased physical activity, low body mass index, earlier menopause, decreased vitamin D synthesis in the fibrotic skin, and involvement of the intestinal tract and kidneys that may impair calcium metabolism. Moreover, even if most patients usually are not exposed to corticosteroids, some manifestations of disease, such as interstitial lung disease, arthritis, myositis, and acute pericarditis, are treated commonly with corticosteroid therapy. In the same way, cyclophosphamide, which is prescribed frequently to patients who have SSc, has been associated with premature ovarian failure [102].

A review of the literature does not allow definitive conclusions about an association between SSc and decreased BMD, or whether clinical features of SSc (eg, disease duration, extent of cutaneous involvement, internal organ involvement, subcutaneous calcinosis) are related directly to osteoporosis risk. Most investigations are retrospective, case-control studies that involved small samples with an insufficient power to detect variables that have a real relationship with a reduced BMD. For example, Di Munno and colleagues [103] showed that patients who had diffuse scleroderma and longer disease duration had lower BMD values, without correlation between BMD and body mass index. Conversely, Da Silva and colleagues [104] and Neuman and colleagues [105] found no differences between diffuse and limited disease. Frediani and colleagues [106] did not find any influence of disease duration on bone loss. Sampaio-Barros and colleagues [107] found that body mass index was the main variable that influenced BMD in a study of 61 women who had SSc. In the same way, internal organ involvement has been regarded as a factor that influences BMD values by some investigators [104], but not by others [103]. These discrepancies could be considered to result from patient selection bias, because the most severe disease is more likely to be influenced by other risk factors for osteoporosis, such as inactivity, poor nutritional state, chronic renal failure, and medications (corticosteroids and cyclophosphamide).

In the attempt to find an altered bone metabolism in patients who have SSc, some studies have addressed this issue by studying bone markers. Most of them did not show changes in calcium metabolism or alterations in bone markers, even in patients who had subcutaneous calcinosis. The only bone marker that was reported to be increased was the urinary pyridinium crosslinks [108]; however, it is still debated whether this result is related to a systemic impairment of collagen turnover and fibrosis rather than to increased bone resorption.

Longitudinal studies probably will be able to confirm the association between SSc and low bone mass, and allow clarification about whether the disease itself actually is related to an increased risk for osteoporosis.

Psoriatic arthritis

Differently from RA, studies about skeletal involvement in patients who have psoriatic arthritis (PsA) are scanty, probably because osteoporosis is a less frequently recognized feature in these subjects. Patients with axial involvement have been included in studies of patients who have AS [78,93,94], without reported differences in comparison with other axial SspAs. With regard to oligo/polyarthritic subsets, PsA is believed to be associated with less severe periarticular bone loss than is RA, as reported by radiological studies on patients with established disease [109]. Nevertheless, a recent study that used DXA to quantify periarticular BMD in patients who had early disease showed no differences in periarticular bone loss in comparison with patients who had RA, even if there was no association between the degree of periarticular bone loss and measures of joint inflammation in patients who had PsA [110].

Few studies have investigated generalized osteoporosis in PsA. Nolla and colleagues [111] found no difference in lumbar and femoral neck BMD in 52 patients who had peripheral PsA compared with controls. Opposite results were achieved by Frediani and colleagues who studied 186 patients who had nonaxial PsA [112]. In this study, the prevalence of osteoporosis was 11% in young women, 47% in postmenopausal women, and 29% in men. Bone loss was more evident at the lumbar level in young women, whereas a reduced femoral neck BMD was detectable only in postmenopausal subjects. Besides well-recognized risk factors for osteoporosis, such as age, years since menopause, and body mass index, the only variable that was related specifically to disease that was predictive of osteoporosis risk was a disability index that is related to articular function (HAQ score).

Polymyalgia rheumatica

Polymyalgia rheumatica (PMR) is an inflammatory disease that affects the elderly population and is treated commonly with corticosteroids. Some studies on patients who have PMR were designed to address the effects on bone metabolism that are exerted by low-dose corticosteroids. But the disease itself seems to alter bone turnover, which causes bone loss early in the disease, before treatment. Dolan and colleagues [113] showed increased levels of resorption markers that correlated with pretreatment disease activity as measured by erythrocyte sedimentation rate and serum interleukin-6, which suggested an effect of systemic inflammation on bone turnover. Patients with a higher acute-phase response at onset had reduced spine BMD before the treatment and a greater bone loss at 1 year. Moreover, by 24 months, as the steroid treatment was reduced or stopped, bone mass improved. Another longitudinal study showed different patterns of bone loss in patients who had PMR, with a faster BMD decrease in regions that contain substantial amounts of trabecular bone and a slower and progressive bone loss at cortical sites [114].

After considering these results, it seems difficult to distinguish the effects of corticosteroids from those of the disease. Even if the degree of inflammation at presentation suggests a role for the disease severity on the development of osteoporosis, it is likely that steroid treatment is the main determinant of bone loss in these patients, taking into account the short time that usually elapses between the onset of PMR and the start of steroid treatment.

Epidemiology of osteoporosis in osteoarthritis

Osteoporosis and OA are the two most common musculoskeletal age-related disorders that may coexist in the same elderly population; however, the potential relationship between these two diseases is controversial and is not understood completely. An inverse association between osteoporosis and OA has been described extensively in the past.

More than 30 years ago some orthopedic surgeons reported on the absence of osteoarthritic changes in excised femoral heads from subjects with hip fractures [115]. These findings demonstrated that hip fractures were more frequent in patients who had the lowest BMD, whereas abnormally high BMD values were found among patients who had OA. This observation was supported further by the description of an increase in BMD at the spine in women who had lumbar spine OA, particularly with osteophytosis [116,117]. In the past, significant differences in terms of anthropometric and skin-fold characteristics were noted between women who had symptomatic postmenopausal osteoporosis and women who had generalized OA [118]. Osteoporotic women were shorter, more slender, and had less fat, muscle girth, and strength, whereas women who had OA, although of comparable age and skeletal size, were more obese and had more fat, muscle mass, and strength. These findings supported the idea that OA and osteoporosis are two different disease entities and are not simple phenomena of aging.

Following this hypothesis, early studies suggested an inverse relationship between the risk for generalized OA and primary osteoporosis. Analyzing 36 publications from 1972 up to 1996, Dequeker and colleagues [119] found a significant increase in bone mass or BMD in patients who had OA compared with age- and sex-matched controls; a correction for anthropometric characteristics (eg, body weight) did not change the results in most studies. Nevertheless, no increase in BMD was found in eight studies. Differences in patient and control selections (ie, the reference population) could explain, at least in part, these controversial reports; differences concerning the measuring site, the techniques of bone mass measurement, and the expression of the results could be important factors for this discrepancy [119].

A higher BMD at skeletal sites that were different from those involved with OA was reported for the hip, knee, hand, and lumbar spine OA in large epidemiologic studies [120–124]. Results from the Chingford population survey demonstrated that women who had OA at different sites (hands, knees, lumbar spine) had significantly higher bone density than did controls at the lumbar spine and hip [120]. In the cross-sectional study of osteoporotic fractures, elevations in BMD were greatest in the femoral neck of hips with OA, in women who had bilateral hip OA, and in women who had hip osteophytes. These findings were consistent with a role for elevated BMD in the pathogenesis of hip OA [121]. These results were confirmed in the Rotterdam study. Examining a population of men and women, Burger and colleagues [125] found that radiographic hip and knee OA was associated with significantly increased BMD ($\sim$3%–8%). This increase was demonstrated according to the number of affected sites and the Kellgren score. Radiographic OA also was associated with significantly elevated bone loss at the hip with age and it seemed to be independent of lower limb disability, which suggested a more pronounced difference in BMD earlier in life. Similar higher rates of bone loss were seen with radiographic OA of the knee in women only. Furthermore, in a twin study, Antoniades and colleagues [126] confirmed an inverse relationship between OA and osteoporosis at the OA-affected hip, but they did not find a clear association between hip OA and BMD at the contralateral site, lumbar spine, or total body. The latter findings suggest that the greater increase in BMD in osteoarthritic subjects that was seen in previous studies of unrelated populations probably is due, in part, to genetic factors that are shared by hip OA and high bone mass. They also suggest that local changes in BMD may be a component of the disease process in hip OA.

In contrast to studies on lower extremity OA, many studies that examined OA of the hand and BMD have not shown consistently similar data. Some showed higher BMD among those who had hand OA [120,124,125], whereas others failed to see such an association. [127,128]. The Rancho Bernardo study investigated the relationship between symptomatic hand OA and BMD in a community-dwelling, ambulatory population of men and women that was older than the age of 50 [129]. In this study, women who had clinically diagnosed hand OA had significantly lower BMD at the hip, whereas there was no consistent significant association between hand OA and BMD among men. These results, together with previous data, support the hypothesis that the apparent inverse relationship between OA and osteoporosis may be related to weight-bearing joints, whereas hand OA might represent another spectrum of the disease that is influenced more by genetics.

Early cross-sectional studies also explored whether the increase in bone mass had any influence on the rates of osteoporotic fractures. A large case-control study of femoral neck fractures from the Mediterranean Osteoporosis Study found that patients who were diagnosed previously with OA were protected from hip fractures by 40% in men and by 60% in women [130]. This association with protection from fracture at any joint in subjects who have OA was confirmed in another population-based case-control study [131]. Moreover, Marcelli and colleagues [124] showed that the severity of OA of the hand correlated positively with bone mass in elderly women, and that women with a higher score of hand OA reported a history of osteoporotic fracture more rarely. Another large epidemiologic study failed to find an association between fracture in any joint and OA, despite the significant increase in BMD in subjects who had OA [132]. The investigators concluded that lack of evidence for reduced fractures might have been due to subjects' postural instability and tendency to fall. Similarly, early results from the Chingford study failed to show a cross-sectional association of forearm and spine fracture with knee and hand OA, but it demonstrated an increased risk for fracture in subjects who had hip OA [133]. Finally, the more recent report from the Study of Osteoporotic Fracture showed that despite having increased BMD, subjects who had hip OA did not have a reduced risk for vertebral fractures [134]. Taken together, these data indicate that patients who have OA should not be considered to be at a lower risk for fracture than is the general population.

The relationship between BMD, osteoporotic fractures, and OA became more complex after results were obtained from more recent epidemiologic studies. In the Framingham cohort longitudinal study, Zhang and colleagues [135] showed that a higher BMD decreased the risk for progression of the disease in the knee (according to Kellgren-Lawrence radiological score) during the follow-up period, but increased the risk for incident radiographic knee OA (defined by osteophytes) in older women. Conversely, among women who had established knee OA, those with low BMD exhibited more rapid progression of radiographic changes than did those with high BMD who lost bone more slowly. These findings were confirmed in a prospective study of 830 middle-aged women from the city of Chingford, United Kingdom [136]. BMD measurements of the lumbar spine and hip as well as radiographs of the knees and hands were performed at baseline; knee radiographs were repeated after 48 months. Baseline BMD at the spine and hip was significantly higher in women who developed incident knee osteophytes 4 years later. More importantly, high BMD was associated with the development of knee osteophytes, but not with joint space narrowing; women who had a fracture during the follow-up period decreased the risk for developing incident knee osteophytes by about 70%, independent of baseline BMD. This evidence indicates that in this population of women, a fracture during the study seemed to protect against incident knee osteophytes irrespective of BMD status; this suggests a possible common role of bone remodeling and repair in the early manifestation of OA. A cross-sectional French study of 559 postmenopausal women (>60 years) investigated the relationship between spine OA and vertebral fracture [137]. Despite a higher BMD, women who had spine OA did not have a reduced risk for fracture. More importantly, disc narrowing was associated with a significant increase in vertebral fracture risk, and this risk increased with the severity of disc narrowing. Recently, the Rotterdam prospective, population-based study added information on the relationship between incident vertebral and nonvertebral fracture and OA [138]. In a sample of 2773 subjects with prevalent radiographic OA of the knee, there was a positive relationship between OA and increased fracture risk. This association seemed to be driven by the presence of osteophytes, rather than by the presence of joint space narrowing. In particular, after adjustment for potential confounding factors, including parameters of postural stability, the relative risks for incident vertebral and nonvertebral fractures in the presence of knee OA were 2 and 1.5, respectively, independent of BMD. A potential explanation for the increased fracture risk in cases of knee OA is that, although these subjects have increased BMD, their bone is of inferior quality at the local level (subchondral trabecular bone of the osteoarthritic knee) and at the systemic level, with generalized altered bone quality and mechanical properties. The fact that the positive association between localized OA and fracture risk is observed especially with the presence of osteophytes supports the hypothesis that an altered bone remodeling (in particular bone formation) is responsible for knee OA and an increase in fragility fractures.

In conclusion, for 3 decades studies have been exploring potential relationships between OA and primary osteoporosis. The evidence for an association with osteoporosis is stronger for large joint OA than for hand OA or primary generalized OA. Although many findings suggest an inverse association between osteoporosis and OA, other data indicate that the two processes are not mutually exclusive and that the prevalence of osteoporosis in the population that has OA may be similar to that seen in the general population. More recent data have shown that the relationship between OA, BMD, and fractures is much more complex than was recognized in the past. Many studies have analyzed the relationship between peripheral OA and osteoporotic fractures, with an increased risk for fracture, no change, or a decreased risk. The discrepancies between studies on fractures in OA may be caused by the site of OA, patient selection, or the method of OA assessment (self-reported or radiographs) that differed from study to study.

Different mechanisms, such as genetic factors [126,139], common risk factors, role of subchondral bone in cartilage damage, and growth factors, are involved in the pathogenesis of OA at different joints [140]. Some evidence indicates that periarticular and systemic changes in the bone architecture, including marked increase in bone turnover [141] and in local factors (ie, IGF-1 and transforming growth factor β), may play a role in altering bone repair, bone quality, and bone strength [142–144]. The challenges are to determine the influences of various biochemical, cellular, and structural forces on bone remodeling and metabolism to increase our understanding of the causes of OA, and, in turn, to design effective management strategies for OA and osteoporosis.

Summary

Much work has been directed at establishing the impact of osteoporosis and related fragility fractures in rheumatic diseases. Several cross-sectional studies reported that disability and reduced motility that are due to functional impairment are among the most important determinants of bone loss in different rheumatic diseases. At the same time, longitudinal studies have confirmed the detrimental effect of uncontrolled disease activity on bone density. In this perspective, the suppression of inflammation probably remains the main concern when considering treatment options. Besides these variables, pharmacologic agents that are used commonly in the treatment of these conditions probably have an adjunctive effect on bone loss in rheumatic patients. Large epidemiologic studies have demonstrated clearly that patients who have RA, SLE, or AS are at an increased risk for fragility fractures. Further studies are required to investigate the effective impact of osteoporosis and fragility fractures in other rheumatic diseases, and to define the relationship between OA and osteoporosis. A better appreciation of the impact and mechanisms of osteoporosis in rheumatic diseases by rheumatologists represents a clinical challenge; however, a greater understanding of this frequent complication will improve the quality of health care and the lives of patients who have rheumatic diseases.

References

[1] Solomon DH, Katz JN, Jacobs JP, et al. Management of glucocorticoid induced osteoporosis in rheumatoid arthritis. Arthritis Rheum 2002;46:3136–42.

[2] Barwell R. Diseases of joints. London: Hardwicke; 1865.

[3] Deodhar AA, Woolf AD. Bone mass measurement and bone metabolism in rheumatoid arthritis: a review. Br J Rheumatol 1996;35:309–22.

[4] Sinigaglia L, Nervetti A, Mela Q, et al. A multicenter cross-sectional study on bone mineral density in rheumatoid arthritis. J Rheumatol 2000;27:2582–9.

[5] Haugeberg G, Uhlig T, Falch JA, et al. Bone mineral density and frequency of osteoporosis in female patients with rheumatoid arthritis. Arthritis Rheum 2000;43:522–30.

[6] Stafford L, Bleasel J, Giles A, et al. Androgen deficiency and bone mineral density in men with rheumatoid arthritis. J Rheumatol 2000;27:2786–90.

[7] Tengstrand B, Hafstrom I. Bone mineral density in men with rheumatoid arthritis is associated with erosive disease and sulfasalazine treatment but not with sex hormones. J Rheumatol 2002;29:2299–305.

[8] Haugeberg G, Uhlig T, Falch JA, et al. Reduced bone mineral density in male rheumatoid arthritis patients. Arhritis Rheum 2000;43:2776–84.

[9] Sambrook PN, Eisman JA, Champion GD, et al. Determinants of axial bone loss in rheumatoid rrthritis. Arthritis Rheum 1987;30:721–7.

[10] Madsen OR, Sorensen OH, Egsmose C. Bone quality and bone mass as assessed by quantitative ultrasound and dual energy X-ray absorptiometry in women with rheumatoid arthritis: relationship with quadriceps strength. Ann Rheum Dis 2002;61:325–9.

[11] Hakkinen A, Sokka T, Kotaniemi A, et al. A randomized two year study of the effects of dynamic strength training on muscle strength, disease activity, functional capacity and bone mineral density in early rheumatoid arthritis. Arthritis Rheum 2001;44:515–22.

[12] Hansen M, Florescu A, Stoltenberg M, et al. Bone loss in rheumatoid arthritis. Influence of disease activity, duration of the disease, functional capacity and corticoid treatment. Scand J Rheumatol 1996;25:367–76.

[13] Als OS, Gotfredsen A, Riis B, et al. Are disease duration and degree of functional impairment determinants of bone loss in rheumatoid arthritis? Ann Rheum Dis 1985;44:406–11.

[14] Shawe D, Hesp R, Gumpel JM, et al. Physical activity as a determinant of bone conservation in the radial diaphysis in rheumatoid arthritis. Ann Rheum Dis 1993;52:579–81.

[15] Sambrook PN, Eisman JA, Yeates MG, et al. Osteoporosis in rheumatoid arthritis: safety of low-dose corticosteroids. Ann Rheum Dis 1986;45:950–3.

[16] Leboff MS, Wade JP, Mackowiak S, et al. Low-dose prednisone does not affect calcium homeostasis or bone density in postmenopausal women with rheumatoid arthritis. J Rheumatol 1991;18:339–44.

[17] Laan RFJM, Van Riel PLCM, Van Earning LJTH, et al. Vertebral osteoporosis in rheumatoid arthritis patients: effect of low-dose prednisolone therapy. Br J Rheumatol 1992;31:91–6.

[18] Hall GM, Spector TD, Griffin AJ, et al. The effect of rheumatoid arthritis and steroid therapy on bone density in postmenopausal women. Arthritis Rheum 1993;36:1510–6.

[19] Shibuya K, Hagino H, Morio Y, et al. Cross-sectional and longitudinal study of osteoporosis in patients with rheumatoid arthritis. Clin Rheumatol 2002;21:150–8.

[20] Sambrook P, Raj A, Hunter D, et al. Osteoporosis with low-dose corticosteroids: contribution of underlying disease effects and discriminatory ability of ultrasound versus bone densitometry. J Rheumatol 2001;28:1063–7.

[21] Lane NE, Pressman AR, Star VL, et al. Rheumatoid arthritis and bone mineral density in elderly women. J Bone Min Res 1995;20:257–63.

[22] Van Staa TP, Leufkens HGM, Cooper C. The epidemiology of corticosteroid-induced osteoporosis: a meta-analysis. Oteoporos Int 2002;13:777–87.

[23] Ton FN, Gunawardene C, Lee H, et al. Effects of low-dose prednisone on bone metabolism. J Bone Min Res 2005;20:464–70.

[24] Di Munno O, Mazzantini M, Sinigaglia L, et al. Effect of low-dose methotrexate on bone density in women with rheumatoid arthritis: results from a multicenter cross-sectional study. J Rheumatol 2004;31:1305–9.

[25] Haugeberg G, Orstavik RE, Uhlig T, et al. Bone loss in patients with rheumatoid arthritis. Arthritis Rheum 2002;46:1720–8.

[26] Shenstone BD, Mahmoud A, Woodward R, et al. Longitudinal bone mineral density changes in early rheumatoid arthritis. Br J Rheumatol 1994;33:541–5.

[27] Gough AKS, Lilley J, Eyre S, et al. Generalised bone loss in patients with early rheumatoid arthritis. Lancet 1994;344:23–7.

[28] Kalla AA, Meyers OL, Chalton D, et al. Increased metacarpal bone mass following 18 months of slow-acting antirheumatic drugs for rheumatoid arthritis. Br J Rheumatol 1991;30:91–100.

[29] Dolan AL, Moniz C, Abraha H, et al. Does active treatment of rheumatoid arthritis limit disease-associated bone loss? Rheumatol 2002;41:1047–51.

[30] Quinn M. The effect of TNF blockade on bone loss in early rheumatoid arthritis. Arthritis Rheum 2002;46(Suppl):S519.

[31] Sambrook PN. The skeleton in rheumatoid arthritis: common mechanisms for bone erosion and osteoporosis? J Rheumatol 2000;27:2541–2.

[32] Lodder MC, de Jong Z, Kostense PJ, et al. Bone mineral density in patients with rheumatoid arthritis: relation between disease severity and low bone mineral density. Ann Rheum Dis 2004;63:1576–80.

[33] Forsblad d'Elia H, Larsen A, Waltbrand E, et al. Radiographic joint destruction in postmenopausal rheumatoid arthritis is strongly associated with generalised osteoporosis. Ann Rheum Dis 2003;62:617–23.

[34] Forslind K, Keller C, Svensson B, et al. Reduced bone mineral density in early rheumatoid arthritis is associated with radiological joint damage at baseline and after two years in women. J Rheumatol 2003;30:2590–6.

[35] Gough A, Sambrook PN, Devlin J, et al. Osteoclastic activation is the principal mechanism leading to secondary osteoporosis in rheumatoid arthritis. J Rheumatol 1998;25:1282–9.

[36] Garnero P, Landewé R, Boers M, et al. Association of baseline levels of markers of bone and cartilage degradation with long-term progression of joint damage in patients with early rheumatoid arthritis. Arthritis Rheum 2002;46:2847–56.

[37] Lodder MC, Haugeberg G, Lems WF, et al. Radiographic damage associated with low bone mineral density and vertebral deformities in rheumatoid arthritis: the Oslo-Truro-Amsterdam (OSTRA) Collaborative Study. Arthritis Rheum 2003;49:209–15.

[38] Hooyman JR, Melton LJ, Nelson AM, et al. Fractures after rheumatoid arthritis: a population-based study. Arthritis Rheum 1984;27:1353–61.

[39] Peel NFA, Moore DJ, Barrington NA, Bax DE, Eastell R. Risk of vertebral fracture and relationship to bone mineral density in steroid treated Rheumatoid Arthritis. Ann Rheum Dis 1995;54:801–6.

[40] Orstavik RE, Haugeberg G, Mowinckel P, et al. Vertebral deformities in rheumatoid arthritis. Arch Intern Med 2004;164:420–5.

[41] Cooper C, Coupland C, Mitchell M. Rheumatoid arthritis, corticosteroid therapy and hip fracture. Ann Rheum Dis 1995;54:49–52.

[42] Huusko TM, Korpela M, Karppi P, et al. Threefold increased risk of hip fractures with rheumatoid arthritis in central Finland. Ann Rheum Dis 2001;60:521–2.

[43] Orstavik RE, Haugeberg G, Uhlig T, et al. Self reported non-vertebral fractures in rheumatoid arthritis and population based controls: incidence and relationship with bone mineral density and clinical variables. Ann Rheum Dis 2004;63:177–82.

[44] Michel BA, Bloch D, Wolfe F, et al. Fractures in rheumatoid arthritis: an evaluation of associated risk factor. J Rheumatol 1993;20:1666–9.

[45] Orstavik RE, Haugeberg G, Uhlig T, et al. Vertebral deformities in 229 female patients with Rheumatoid Arthritis: associations with clinical variables and bone mineral density. Arthritis Rheum 2003;49:355–60.

[46] Kaz Kaz H, Johnson D, Kerry S, et al. Fall-related risk factors and osteoporosis in women with rheumatoid arthritis. Rheumatol 2004;43:1267–71.

[47] Jamison M, Neuberger GB, Miller PA. Correlates of falls and fear of falling among adults with rheumatoid arthritis. Arthritis Rheum 2003;49:673–80.

[48] Haugeberg G, Orstavik RE, Uhlig T, et al. Clinical decision rules in rheumatoid arthritis: do they identify patients at high risk for osteoporosis? Testing clinical criteria in a population based cohort of patients with rheumatoid arthritis recruited from the Oslo Rheumatoid Arthritis Register. Ann Rheum Dis 2002;61:1085–9.

[49] Sinigaglia L, Varenna M, Binelli L, et al. Bone mass in systemic lupus erythematosus. Clin Exp Rheumatol 2000;18(Suppl 2)19:S27–34.

[50] Dhillon VB, Davies MC, Hall ML, et al. Assessment of the effect of oral corticosteroids on bone mineral density in systemic lupus erythematosus: a preliminary study with dual energy X ray absorptiometry. Ann Rheum Dis 1990;49:624–6.

[51] Houssiau FA, Lefebvre C, Depresseux G, et al. Trabecular and cortical bone loss in systemic lupus erythematosus. Br J Rheumatol 1996;35:244–7.

[52] Sels F, Dequeker J, Verwilghen J, et al. SLE and osteoporosis: dependence and/or independence on glucocorticoids. Lupus 1996;5:89–92.

[53] Kalla AA, Fataar AB, Jessop SJ, et al. Loss of trabecular bone mineral density in systemic lupus erythematosus. Arthritis Rheum 1993;12:1726–34.

[54] Formiga F, Moga I, Nolla JM, et al. Loss of bone mineral density in premenopausal women with systemic lupus erythematosus. Ann Rheum Dis 1995;54:274–6.

[55] Li EK, Tam LS, Young RP, et al. Loss of bone mineral density in Chinese premenopausal women with systemic lupus erythematosus treated with corticosteroids. Br J Rheumatol 1998;37:405–10.

[56] Pineau CA, Urowitz MB, Fortin D, et al. Osteoporosis in systemic lupus erythematosus: factors associated with referral for bone mineral density studies, prevalence of osteoporosis and factors associated with reduced bone density. Lupus 2004;13:436–41.

[57] Lee C, Alamagor A, Dunlop DD, et al. Disease damage and low bone mineral density: an analysis of women with systemic lupus erythematosus ever and never receiving corticosteroids. Rheumatol 2006;45:53–60.

[58] Pons F, Peris P, Guanabens N, et al. The effect of systemic lupus erythematosus and long-term steroid therapy on bone mass in premenopausal women. Br J Rheumatol 1995;34:742–6.

[59] Kipen Y, Buchbinder R, Strauss BJG, et al. Prevalence of reduced bone mineral density in systemic lupus arythematosus and the role of glucocorticoids. J Rheumatol 1997;24:1922–9.

[60] Sinigaglia L, Varenna M, Binelli L, et al. Determinants of bone mass in systemic lupus erythematosus: a cross-sectional study on premenopausal women. J Rheumatol 1999;26:1280–4.

[61] Yee C-S, Crabtree N, Skan J, et al. Prevalence and predictors of fragility fractures in systemic lupus erythematosus. Ann Rheum Dis 2005;64:111–3.

[62] Uaratanawong S, Deesomchoke U, Lertmaharit S, et al. Bone mineral density in premen-opausal women with systemic lupus erythematosus. J Rheumatol 2003;30:2365–8.

[63] Lilleby V, Lien G, Froslie KF, et al. Frequency of osteopenia in children and young adults with childhood-onset systemic lupus erythematosus. Arthritis Rheum 2005;52:2051–9.

[64] Petri M. Musculoskeletal complications of systemic lupus erythematosus in the Hopkins Lupus Cohort: an update. Arthritis Care Res 1995;8:137–45.

[65] Mok CC, Mak A, Ma KM. Bone mineral density in postmenopausal Chinese patients with systemic lupus erythematosus. Lupus 2005;14:106–12.

[66] Formiga F, Nolla JM, Moga I, et al. Sequential study of bone mineral density in patients with systemic lupus erythematosus [letter]. Ann Rheum Dis 1996;55:857.

[67] Hansen M, Halberg P, Kollerup G, et al. Bone metabolism in patients with systemic lupus erythematosus. Scand J Rheumatol 1998;27:197–206.

[68] Kipen Y, Briganti E, Strauss B, et al. Three year follow up of bone mineral density change in premenopausal women with systemic lupus erythematosus. J Rheumatol 1999;26:310–7.

[69] Trapani S, Civinini R, Ermini M, et al. Osteoporosis in juvenile systemic lupus erythema-tosus: a longitudinal study on the effects of steroids on bone mineral density. Rheumatol Int 1998;18:45–9.

[70] Teichmann J, Lange U, Strackc H, et al. Bone metabolism and bone mineral density of sys-temic lupus erythematosus at the time of diagnosis. Rheumatol Int 1999;18:137–40.

[71] Formiga F, Nolla JM, Mitjavila F, et al. Bone mineral density and hormonal status in men with systemic lupus erythematosus. Lupus 1996;5:623–6.

[72] Bultink IEM, Lems WF, Kostense PJ, et al. Prevalence and risk factors for low bone min-eral density and vertebral fractures in patients with systemic lupus erythematosus. Arthritis Rheum 2005;54:2044–50.

[73] Borba VZC, Matos PG, Da Silva Viana PR, et al. High prevalence of vertebral deformity in premenopausal systemic lupus erythematosus patients. Lupus 2005;14:529–33.

[74] Ramsey-Goldman R, Dunn JE, Huang CF, et al. Frequency of fractures in women with sys-temic lupus erythematosus. Arthritis Rheum 1999;42:882–90.

[75] Hanson CA, Shagrin JW, Duncan H. Vertebral osteoporosis in ankylosing spondylitis. Clin Orthop 1971;74:59–64.

[76] Spencer DG, Park WM, Dick HM, et al. Radiological manifestations in 200 patients with ankylosing spondylitis: correlation with clinical features and HLA B27. J Rheumatol 1979; 6:305–15.

[77] Will R, Palmer R, Bhalla AK, et al. Osteoporosis in early ankylosing spondylitis: a primary event? Lancet 1989;2:1483–5.

[78] Donnelly S, Doyle DV, Denton A, et al. Bone mineral density and vertebral compression fracture rates in ankylosing spondylitis. Ann Rheum Dis 1994;53:117–21.

[79] Mitra D, Elvins DM, Speden DJ, et al. The prevalence of vertebral fractures in mild an-kylosing spondylitis and their relationship to bone mineral density. Rheumatol 2000;39: 85–9.

[80] Lee LYS, Schlotzhauer T, Ott SM, et al. Skeletal status of men with early and late ankylos-ing spondylitis. Am J Med 1997;103:233–41.

[81] Bronson WD, Walker SE, Hillman LS, et al. Bone mineral density and biochemical markers of bone metabolism in ankylosing spondylitis. J Rheumatol 1998;25:929–35.

[82] Reid DM, Nicoll JJ, Kennedy NS, et al. Bone mass in ankylosing spondylitis. J Rheumatol 1986;13:932–5.

[83] Mullaji AB, Upadhyay SS, Ho EK. Bone mineral density in ankylosing spondylitis. DEXA comparison of control subjects with mild and advanced cases. J Bone Joint Surg Br 1994;76: 660–5.

[84] Devogelaer J-P, Maldague B, Malghem J, et al. Appendicular and vertebral bone mass in ankylosing spondylitis. Arthritis Rheum 1992;35:1062–7.

[85] Lange U, Kluge A, Strunk J, et al. Ankylosing spondylitis and bone mineral density. What is the ideal tool for measurement? Rheumatol Int 2005;26(2):115–20.

[86] Karberg K, Zochling J, Sieper J, et al. Bone loss is detected more frequently in patients with ankylosing spondylitis with syndesmophytes. J Rheumatol 2005;32:1290–8.

[87] Gilgil E, Kacar C, Tuncer T, et al. The association of syndesmophytes with vertebral bone mineral density in patients with ankylosing spondylitis. J Rheumatol 2005;32:292–4.

[88] Toussirot E, Michel F, Wendling D. Bone density, ultrasound measurements and body composition in early ankylosing spondylitis. Rheumatol 2001;40:882–8.

[89] Juanola X, Mateo L, Nolla J-M, et al. Bone mineral density in women with ankylosing spondylitis. J Rheumatol 2000;27:1028–31.

[90] Speden DJ, Calin AI, Ring FJ, et al. Bone mineral density, calcaneal ultrasound, and bone turnover markers in women with ankylosing spondylitis. J Rheumatol 2002;29:516–21.

[91] Grisar J, Bernecker PM, Aringer M, et al. Ankylosing spondylitis, psoriatic arthritis, and reactive arthritis show increased bone resorption, but differ with regard to bone formation. J Rheumatol 2002;29:1430–6.

[92] Gratacos J, Collado A, Pons F, et al. Significant loss of bone mass in patients with early, active ankylosing spondylitis. Arthritis Rheum 1999;42:2319–24.

[93] Maillefert JF, Aho LS, El Maghraoui A, et al. Changes in bone density in patients with ankylosing spondylitis: a two-year follow-up study. Osteoporos Int 2001;12:605–9.

[94] El Maghraoui A, Borderie D, Cherruau B, et al. Osteoporosis, body composition, and bone turnover in ankylosing spondylitis. J Rheumatol 1999;26:2205–9.

[95] Cooper C, Carbone L, Michet CJ, et al. Fracture risk in patients with ankylosing spondylitis: a population based study. J Rheumatol 1994;21:1877–82.

[96] Ralston SH, Urquhart GDK, Brzeski M, et al. Prevalence of vertebral compression fractures due to osteoporosis in ankylosing spondylitis. BMJ 1990;300:563–5.

[97] Thorngren KG, Liedberg E, Aspelin P. Fractures of the thoracic and lumbar spine in ankylosing spondylitis. Arch Orthop Traumat Surg 1981;98:101–7.

[98] Murray GC, Persellin RH. Cervical fracture complicating in ankylosing spondylitis: a report of eight cases and review of the literature. Am J Med 1981;70:1033–41.

[99] Grisolia A, Bell R, Peltier L. Fractures and dislocations of the spine complicating ankylosing spondylitis. J Bone Joint Surg Am 1967;49:339–44.

[100] Sivri A, Killinc S, Gökce-Kutsal Y, et al. Bone mineral density in ankylosing spondylitis. Clin Rheumatol 1996;15:51–4.

[101] Baek HJ, Kang SW, Lee JY, et al. Osteopenia in men with mild and severe ankylosing spondylitis. Rheumatol Int 2005;26:30–4.

[102] Mok CC, Lau CS, Wong RWS. Risk factors for ovarian failure in patients with systemic lupus erythematosus receiving cyclophosphamide therapy. Arthritis Rheum 1998;41:831–7.

[103] Di Munno O, Mazzantini M, Massei P, et al. Reduced bone mass and normal calcium metabolism in systemic sclerosis with and without calcinosis. Clin Rheumatol 1995;14:407–12.

[104] Da Silva HC, Szejnfeld VL, Assis LS, et al. Study of bone density in systemic scleroderma. Rev Assoc Med Bras 1997;43:40–6.

[105] Neuman K, Wallace K, Metzger A. Osteoporosis. Less than expected in patients with scleroderma. J Rheumatol 2000;27:1822–3.

[106] Frediani B, Baldi F, Falsetti P, et al. Clinical determinants of bone mass and bone ultrasonometry in patients with systemic sclerosis. Clin Exp Rheum 2004;22:313–8.

[107] Sampaio-Barros PD, Costa-Paiva L, Filardi S, et al. Prognostic factors of low bone mineral density in systemic sclerosis. Clin Exp Rheum 2005;23:180–4.

[108] Istok R, Czirjak L, Lukac J, et al. Increased urinary pyridinoline cross-link compounds of collagen in patients with systemic sclerosis and Raynaud's phenomenon. Rheumatology (Oxford) 2001;40:140–6.

[109] Wright V. Psoriatic arthritis: a comparative radiographic study of rheumatoid arthritis and arthritis associated with psoriasis. Ann Rheum Dis 1961;20:123–31.

[110] Harrison BJ, Hutchinson CE, Adams J, et al. Assessing periarticular bone mineral density in patients with early psoriatic arthritis or rheumatoid arthritis. Ann Rheum Dis 2002;61:1007–11.

[111] Nolla JM, Rozadilla A, Gomez-Vaquero C, et al. Bone mineral density in patients with peripheral psoriatic arthritis. Rev Rhum Engl Ed 1999;66:457–61.

[112] Frediani B, Allegri A, Falsetti P, et al. Bone mineral density in patients with psoriatic arthritis. J Rheumatol 2001;28:138–43.

[113] Dolan AL, Moniz C, Dasgupta B, et al. Effects of inflammation and treatment on bone turnover and bone mass in polymyalgia rheumatica. Arthritis Rheum 1997;40:2022–9.

[114] Pearce G, Ryan PFJ, Delmas PD, et al. The deleterious effects of low-dose corticosteroids on bone density in patients with polymyalgia rheumatica. Br J Rheumatol 1998;37:292–9.

[115] Foss MVL, Byers PD. Bone density, osteoarthrosis of the hip and fracture of the upper end of the femur. Ann Rheum Dis 1972;31:259–64.

[116] Jones G, Nguyen T, Sambrook PN, et al. A longitudinal study of the effect of spinal degenerative disease on bone density in the elderly. J Rheumatol 1995;22:932–6.

[117] Liu G, Peacock M, Eilam O, et al. Effect of osteoarthritis in the lumbar spine and hip on bone mineral density and diagnosis of osteoporosis in elderly men and women. Osteoporos Int 1997;7:564–9.

[118] Dequeker J, Goris P, Uytterhoeven R. Osteoporosis and osteoarthritis (osteoarthrosis). Anthropometric distinctions. JAMA 1983;249:1448–51.

[119] Dequeker J, Boonen S, Aerssens J, et al. Inverse relationship osteoarthritis-osteoporosis: what is the evidence? What are the consequences? Br J Rheumatol 1996;35(9):813–8.

[120] Hart D, Mootoosamy I, Doyle D, et al. The relationship between osteoarthritis and osteoporosis in the general population: the Chingford Study. Ann Rheum Dis 1994;53:158–62.

[121] Nevitt M, Lane N, Scott J, et al. Radiographic osteoarthritis of the hip and bone mineral density. Arthritis Rheum 1995;38:907–16.

[122] Hannan MT, Anderson JJ, Zhang Y, et al. Bone mineral density and knee osteoarthritis in elderly men and women. Arthritis Rheum 1993;36:1671–80.

[123] Belmonte-Serrano MA, Bloch A, Lane NE, et al. The relationship between spinal and peripheral osteoarthritis and bone density measurements. J Rheumatol 1993;20:1005–13.

[124] Marcelli C, Favier F, Kotzki P, et al. The relationship between osteoarthritis of the hands, bone mineral density, and osteoporotic fractures in elderly women. Osteoporos Int 1995;5: 382–8.

[125] Burger H, van Daele PLA, Odding E, et al. Association of radiographically evident osteoarthritis with higher bone mineral density and increased bone loss with age: the Rotterdam Study. Arthritis Rheum 1996;39:81–6.

[126] Antoniades L, MacGregor AJ, Matson M, et al. A cotwin control study of the relationship between hip osteoarthritis and bone mineral density. Arthritis Rheum 2000;43:1450–5.

[127] Hochberg M, Lethbridge-Cejku M, Scott W, et al. Appendicular bone mass and osteoarthritis of the hands in women: Data from the Baltimore Longitudinal Study of Aging. J Rheumatol 1994;21:1532–6.

[128] Sowers M, Zobel D, Weissfeld L, et al. Progression of osteoarthritis of the hand and metacarpal bone loss. A twenty-year followup of incident cases. Arthritis Rheum 1991;34:36–42.

[129] Schneider DL, Barrett-Connor E, Morton DJ, et al. Bone mineral density and clinical hand osteoarthritis in elderly men and women: The Rancho Bernardo Study. J Rheumatol 2002, 29:1467–72.

[130] Dequeker J, Johnell O. Osteoarthritis protects against femoral neck fracture: the MEDOS study experience. Bone 1993;14(Suppl 1):S51–6.

[131] Cumming RG, Klineberg RJ. Epidemiological study of the relation between arthritis of the hip and hip fractures. Ann Rheum Dis 1993;52:707–10.

[132] Jones G, Nguyen T, Sambrook PN, et al. Osteoarthritis, bone density, postural stability, and osteoporotic fractures: a population based study. J Rheumatol 1995;22:921–5.

[133] Arden NK, Griffiths GO, Hart DJ, et al. The association between osteoarthritis and osteoporotic fracture: the Chingford Study. Br J Rheumatol 1996;35:1299–304.

[134] Arden NK, Nevitt MC, Lane NE, et al. Osteoarthritis and risk of falls, rates of bone loss, and osteoporotic fractures. Arthritis Rheum 1999;42:1378–85.

[135] Zhang Y, Hannan MT, Chaisson CE, et al. Bone mineral density and risk of incident and progressive radiographic knee osteoarthritis in women: the Framingham Study. J Rheumatol 2000;27:1032–7.

[136] Hart DJ, Cronin C, Daniels M, et al. The relationship of bone density and fracture to incident and progressive radiographic osteoarthritis of the knee: the Chingford Study. Arthritis Rheum 2002;46:92–9.

[137] Sornay-Rendu E, Munoz F, Duboeuf F, et al. Disc space narrowing is associated with an increased vertebral fracture risk in postmenopausal women: the OFELY study. J Bone Miner Res 2004;19:1994–9.

[138] Bergink AP, Van der Klift M, Hofman A, et al. Osteoarthritis of the knee is associated with vertebral and nonvertebral fractures in the elderly: the Rotterdam Study. Arthritis Rheum 2003;49:648–57.

[139] Naganathan V, Zochling J, March L, et al. Peak bone mass is increased in the hip in daughters of women with osteoarthritis. Bone 2002;30:287–92.

[140] Sambrook P, Naganathan V. What is the relationship between osteoarthritis and osteoporosis? Baillieres Clin Rheumatol 1997;11:695–710.

[141] Gilertson EM. Development of periarticular osteophytes in experimentally induced osteoarthritis in the dog. A study using microradiographic, microangiographic, and fluorescent bone-labelling techniques. Ann Rheum Dis 1975;34:12–25.

[142] Radin EL, Rose RM. Role of subchondral bone in the initiation and progression of cartilage damage. Clin Orthop Relat Res 1986;213:34–40.

[143] Dequeker J, Mohan S, Finkelman RD, et al. Generalized osteoarthritis associated with increased insulin-like growth factor types I and II and transforming growth factor beta in cortical bone from the iliac crest. Possible mechanism of increased bone density and protection against osteoporosis. Arthritis Rheum 1993;36:1702–8.

[144] Uchino M, Izumi T, Tominaga T, et al. Growth factor expression in the osteophytes of the human femoral head in osteoarthritis. Clin Orthop Relat Res 2000;377:119–25.

ELSEVIER
SAUNDERS

RHEUMATIC
DISEASE CLINICS
OF NORTH AMERICA

Rheum Dis Clin N Am 32 (2006) 659–680

Genetics and Osteoporosis

Omar M.E. Albagha, MSc, PhD*,
Stuart H. Ralston, MD, FRCP

*Rheumatology Section, Molecular Medicine Centre,
University of Edinburgh School of Molecular and Clinical Medicine,
Western General Hospital, Edinburgh, EH4 2XU, United Kingdom*

Genetic factors play an important role in the pathogenesis of osteoporosis. The importance of genetic factors in regulating susceptibility to osteoporosis is highlighted by the observation that a positive family history of hip fracture is a strong risk factor for low bone mineral density (BMD) and osteoporotic fracture [1,2]. Although fracture is the most important clinical complication of osteoporosis, most studies of genetics have focused on BMD, because this is a highly heritable trait [3–6] and an important clinical predictor of osteoporotic fracture risk [7]. Nonetheless, evidence of significant genetic effects on other key determinants of osteoporotic fracture risk, such as quantitative ultrasound properties of bone [8], femoral neck geometry [8], muscle strength [9], bone turnover markers [10], and body mass index [11], has also been reported. Much less information exists about the heritability of fracture, which is the most important clinical consequence of osteoporosis. Some investigators found little evidence to suggest that fractures are heritable in the elderly [12], whereas other researchers reported that wrist fracture had a significant genetic component with heritability estimates in the range of 25% to 35% [13,14]. Interestingly, these studies showed that susceptibility to wrist fracture appeared to be largely independent of BMD. Other work has shown that the heritability of fracture is high in younger patients but falls off rapidly with age to almost zero in the elderly [15], this would explain the discrepancies between the studies cited earlier. BMD and the other traits mentioned earlier are regulated by multiple genes and their interaction with environmental factors.

* Corresponding author.
E-mail address: omar.albagha@ed.ac.uk (O.M.E. Albagha).

0889-857X/06/$ - see front matter © 2006 Elsevier Inc. All rights reserved.
doi:10.1016/j.rdc.2006.08.001   *rheumatic.theclinics.com*

Genetic approaches to identification of osteoporosis susceptibility genes

Three primary approaches have been implemented in the identification of genes that predispose to osteoporosis: linkage analysis in pedigrees, experimental crosses in model animals, and association studies in human populations. The basic principles of these methods and their use in the identification of genetic loci for susceptibility to osteoporosis are discussed in more detail in this section.

Linkage analysis in pedigrees

Classic linkage analysis in human pedigrees has been used widely and successfully for mapping single-disease genes. The principle of this approach is outlined in Fig. 1, left panel. It involves genotyping family members for a number of polymorphic genetic markers, then looking for evidence of cosegregation of a particular marker with the disease phenotype under a predefined model of inheritance. Genetic markers located close to the disease-causing gene will cosegregate with the phenotype. Linkage is measured by lodscore. For Mendelian diseases, linkage is considered significant when

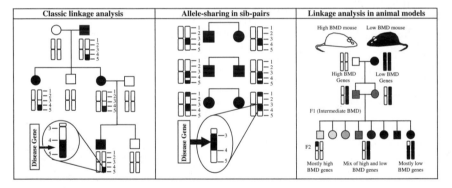

Fig. 1. Genetic approaches used in the identification of osteoporosis susceptibility genes. (*Left panel*) Linkage analysis in pedigrees. **Principle:** Look for cosegregation of a polymorphic marker with the disease in pedigrees. In the provided example markers 4 and 5 are segregating with the disease status, indicating that the disease gene is located between these two markers. **Advantage:** Suitable for mapping single-gene or oligogenic disorders. **Disadvantages:** Requires large multigenerational pedigrees and defined model of inheritance. (*Middle panel*) Allele sharing. **Principle:** Test whether affected relatives share a certain chromosomal region more often than expected by random segregation. In the given example, the region between marker 3 and 4 is shared between all affected sib-pairs, indicating that the disease gene may be located between these two markers. **Advantage:** More suitable for mapping complex disease genes when mode of inheritance cannot be defined. **Disadvantages:** Large number of sib-pairs is required. (*Right panel*) Animal studies. **Principle:** Involve crosses between two different strains of animals. In the given example, a mouse strain with low BMD is crossed with a high-BMD strain, and genetic loci may be identified by analysis of the F2 generation, looking for cosegregation of genetic markers with BMD loci. **Advantage:** Large number of animals may be obtained; breeding program may be controlled. **Disadvantages:** Loci identified may be species-specific; requires animal model for the phenotype under investigation.

the lodscore values exceed 3.0 (odds ratio of linkage against no linkage >1000) and may be excluded when lodscore values are less than −2.0. Suggestive linkage is defined as lodscore values between 2.2 and 3.0. For complex diseases in which linkage studies are generally performed using nonparametric analysis methods, however, the significance thresholds are higher. A lodscore of greater than 3.6 must be obtained for significant linkage [16]. Linkage studies are usually performed on a genome-wide basis using a fixed panel of microsatellite markers that are approximately 10 centimorgans apart. However, over recent years, panels of closely spaced single nucleotide polymorphism (SNP) markers have been developed that offer improved statistical power in performing genome-wide scans for complex diseases [17]. Genome-wide scans using the classic linkage approach have been used successfully to map genetic loci for rare monogenic bone diseases, such as osteoporosis-pseudoglioma syndrome and high bone mass trait [18,19]. However, this approach is less suitable for the study of complex diseases such as osteoporosis or complex traits such as BMD, because of the difficulty of finding multigenerational informative families and unknown mode of inheritance.

Another linkage analysis method for mapping quantitative trait loci (QTLs) and complex disease genes has been developed to tackle the limitation of the classic linkage methods. The analysis is based on allele sharing in sib pairs (see Fig. 1, middle panel). Allele-sharing methods involve testing whether affected relatives inherit a certain chromosomal region more often than would be expected under random Mendelian segregation. This method, in contrast to classic linkage studies, is not affected by locus heterogeneity and does not require construction of a disease model. Therefore, the allele-sharing method has been the most widely used approach for mapping complex disease genes such as osteoporosis. However, the success of this approach is dependent on the availability of a large number of sib-pairs to gain adequate statistical power to detect genes with modest effect. The first genome-wide linkage search to identify QTLs that contribute to the genetic variations of BMD was performed by Devoto and colleagues [20] in families with history of osteoporosis. The authors analyzed the data using two different methods: the classic linkage analysis and allele-sharing methods. Although none of the QTLs identified by the classic linkage approach reached the statistical significance for linkage, several QTLs with suggestive or significant linkage were identified when the data were analyzed using the allele-sharing methods (Table 1). This finding demonstrated that classic linkage analysis is less suitable for mapping complex disease genes.

Another statistical method of performing genome-wide linkage scans was developed by Almasy and Blangero [21], based on variance component linkage analysis. The advantage of this approach is that it allows one to estimate the contribution of possible covariates affecting the phenotype under investigation. When one is studying BMD, the contribution of environmental factors (such as calcium intake, physical activity, smoking, and estrogen use), as well as other important confounding factors such as age, weight,

Table 1
Major quantitative trait loci for bone mineral density identified by linkage analysis in humans

Study	Study design	Statistical approach	Chromosome	Lod score	Phenotype	Gender
Devoto et al (1998) [20]	History of osteoporosis	Allele-sharing	1p36	2.29	FN-BMD	M & F
			2p23-24	2.25	LS-BMD	M & F
			4qter	2.28	FN-BMD	M & F
Niu et al (1999) [117]	Healthy sib-pair	Allele-sharing	2p21-24	2.15	Forearm-BMD	M & F
Koller et al (2000) [118]	Healthy sib-pair	Allele-sharing	1q21-23	3.11	LS-BMD	F
Karasik et al (2002) [119]	Normal Population	Variance component	21q22.2	2.39	TR-BMD	M & F
			21qter	3.14	TR-BMD	M & F
Deng et al (2002) [120]	Proband with low BMD	Variance component	4q31-32	3.08	Spine BMD	M & F
			10q26	2.29	FN-BMD	M & F
			13q33-34	2.43	LS- BMD	M & F
Karasik et al (2003) [121]	Normal population	Variance component	9q22-31	2.71	FN-BMD	F
			12q23-24	3.00	TR-BMD	F
			14q31	2.48	LS-BMD	F
Kammerer et al (2003) [122]	Normal population	Variance component	2p25	3.98	FN-BMD	M
			4p15	4.33	Forearm BMD	M & F
			6q27	2.27	TR-BMD	M & F
			12q24	2.24	Forearm BMD	M & F
			13q14	3.46	TR-BMD	M
			13q14	2.51	FN-BMD	M
Wilson et al (2003) [110]	Dizygotic female twins	Allele sharing	1p36	2.38	Whole body BMD	F
			3p21	2.72	LS-BMD	F
Styrkarsdottir et al (2003) [27]	History of osteoporosis	Allele-sharing	20p12	3.18	FN-BMD	M & F
			20p12	2.89	LS-BMD	M & F

Study	Population	Method	Location	LOD	BMD	Sex
Shen et al (2004) [123]	Normal population + probands with low BMD	Variance component	11q23	3.13	LS-BMD	M & F
			Xq27	4.30	Forearm BMD	M & F
			Xq27	2.57	FN-BMD	M & F
Ralston et al (2005) [26]	History of osteoporosis	Variance component	3q25	2.43	FN-BMD	M
			4q25	2.22	FN-BMD	M
			4q25	2.55	FN-BMD	F
			7p14	2.28	FN-BMD	M
			10q21	4.2	FN-BMD	M
			16p13	2.52	FN-BMD	M
			16q23	2.28	LS-BMD	F
			18p11	2.83	LS-BMD	F
			20q13	3.2	LS-BMD	F
Peacock et al (2005) [124]	Normal population	Allele sharing	1q	3.13	LS-BMD	M
			2p	4.4	LS-BMD	M & F
			2p	2.99	FN-BMD	M
			14p	4.6	LS-BMD	M

Abbreviations: F, females; FN, femoral neck; LS, lumbar spine; M, males; TR, trochanter.

and body mass index, may be included in the variance component analysis. The variance component method has been used by many investigators to perform genome-wide scans to identify QTLs that regulate BMD and other osteoporosis-related phenotypes. Table 1 summarizes the QTLs for BMD regulation identified by various genome-wide linkage studies with significant or suggestive linkage.

Lee and colleagues [22] have recently performed a meta-analysis of 11 previously published genome-wide scans to assess evidence for linkage of BMD across whole genome scan studies. They analyzed the data from approximately 3000 families and found that the region on chromosome 16pter-16p12.3 has the greatest evidence of linkage. An interesting finding to emerge from this meta-analysis is the identification of two chromosomal regions (10p14-q11, 22q12-pter) with evidence for linkage that have not been detected by individual studies. However, the authors used published linkage scores instead of whole genome data, which reduces the statistical power of the study, and the analysis did not take into account the ethnic differences in genetic loci for BMD regulation.

Genome-wide scans for regulation of other osteoporosis-related phenotypes, such as hip geometry and quantitative ultrasound properties of bone, have been reported. Several loci for regulation of various aspects of femoral neck geometry were identified in a linkage study performed by Koller and colleagues [23]. Wilson and colleagues [24] identified two QTLs for quantitative ultrasound of the calcaneus on chromosome 2q33-37 and 4q12-21 in a large twin cohort. Sex-specific QTLs for bone structure at the proximal femur have also been reported [25].

Several important observations have emerged from the linkage studies that have been performed in the field of osteoporosis genetics. It is now clear that most of the loci that regulate BMD do so in a site-specific and gender-specific manner, although a few QTLs have been identified where there are effects in both genders and in BMD at more than one skeletal site. Another feature to emerge from studies that categorized patients by age group is that the loci regulating peak bone mass are probably different from those that regulate BMD in older people [26]. This finding raises the possibility that genes that regulate BMD may differ from those that regulate bone loss, although the evidence in favor of genetic effects on bone loss is very limited. Another important point is that few genome-wide scans have actually identified loci that reach the threshold for genome-wide significance. So far, only one gene for osteoporosis susceptibility has actually been identified by linkage and positional cloning, and this was the bone morphogenetic protein 2 in the isolated population of Iceland [27].

Animal studies

Based on the assumption that key genes regulating BMD are shared across species, linkage studies in model animals provide another approach to the genetic basis of osteoporosis. The principle of this approach is outlined in Fig. 1, right panel. A cross of one inbred mouse strain with high BMD and another with low BMD is usually performed and followed by a brother–sister mating of the F1 animals to generate an F2 strain of animals with variable levels of BMD owing to segregation of the alleles that regulate BMD. A genome-wide scan is performed in the F2 generation to identify QTLs that regulate BMD. The first genome search for QTLs for bone mass regulation in mice was performed by Klein and colleagues [28], who identified 10 genetic loci that were linked to bone mass in female mice and four other loci linked to body weight. Subsequent genome searches by various investigators identified many other QTLs for BMD regulation that are distributed across the mouse chromosomes [29–31]. Gene mapping studies in mice have identified QTLs for other bone phenotypes relevant to osteoporosis, including femoral cross-sectional area [32], trabecular bone volume and microarchitecture [33], and mechanical properties of the mouse femur [34].

Interestingly, QTLs regulating bone phenotypes in mice were found to be gender specific [35,36] and skeletal-site specific [37,38], consistent with the observations reported in humans. Although many QTLs identified are specific to individual mouse strains, replication of some QTLs for BMD regulation between different strains has been reported, suggesting that some of the genetic variants in these loci may be highly conserved. Furthermore, some QTLs for regulation of BMD identified in the mouse show synteny with QTLs identified in humans. An example is the QTL identified on mouse chromosome 4 near the marker D4Mit312 (lodscore = 12.3), which is homologous to the QTL on the human chromosome 1p36 identified by various linkage studies (see Table 1). Because most QTL mapping has been performed in inbred strains, fine mapping attempts to narrow down the QTL have been reported [39], but so far there has been limited success in identifying the causative gene.

A notable exception is the case of a mouse chromosome 11 QTL identified by Klein and colleagues [40]. Here the investigators studied the expression profile for genes in the region using microarray technology. They found that the expression level of *ALOX15* in the DBA2 strain of mice (low BMD strain) was 20-fold greater than the expression level in C57BL/6 mice (high BMD strain), suggesting that *ALOX15* may act as a negative regulator of peak bone mass in mice. Consistent with this hypothesis, *ALOX15* knockout mice had increased BMD. A recent study has also shown that polymorphisms in the human *ALOX15* gene were associated with BMD in postmenopausal Japanese women [41]. The mechanism by which *ALOX15* regulates BMD is still unclear, but some have hypothesized that it may be involved in osteoblast and adipocyte differentiation through activation of the PPAR (peroxisome proliferator-activated receptor) gamma receptor. A recent study has also shown that the human chromosome Xp22 region, which is syntenic to a QTL for BMD regulation identified on mouse chromosome X, may also contain genes that regulate BMD in humans. This finding demonstrates the possibility of transferring loci for BMD regulation between the mouse and the human genomes [42]. In summary, linkage studies in mice have identified many QTLs for BMD regulation. However, further studies are required to identify the genes responsible and to investigate whether these genes are also involved in the pathogenesis of osteoporosis in humans.

Association studies of candidate genes

By far the greatest portion of information on the genes associated with osteoporosis susceptibility comes from association studies in candidate genes. Association studies are based on comparing allele frequency for a polymorphism in or around a candidate gene of interest in a case and control group of individuals. Disease-associated alleles will be overrepresented in affected individuals as compared with controls. Quantitative traits such as BMD may also be investigated by comparing the mean values of the trait in different genotype groups for the polymorphisms under study. The principle of the classic association study is outlined in Fig. 2.

Recently, however, it has become possible to perform association studies on a genome-wide basis by analyzing a large number of closely spaced SNPs spread randomly across the genome [43]. The rationale for these studies is that these SNPs will be in linkage disequilibrium with causal variants in genes that predispose to the disease under study. Genome-wide association

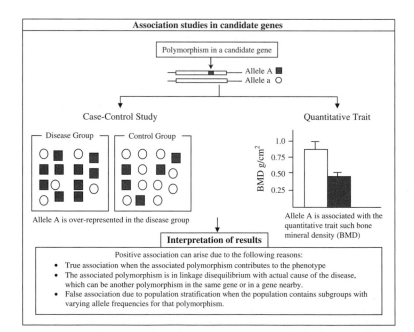

Fig. 2. Using association studies to identify genes for BMD regulation.

studies present a major challenge in terms of statistical analysis, but the very high density of marker panels now available offers the prospect of identifying genes and genomic regions that contribute to complex diseases such as osteoporosis.

The most widely studied candidate genes for BMD regulation include those with an obvious function in bone physiology, such as the vitamin D receptor (*VDR*), the collagen type I alpha 1 (*COLIA1*), and the estrogen receptor alpha gene (*ESR1*). Other candidate genes have been studied in relation to osteoporosis because of their involvement in rare bone disorders affecting BMD regulation, such as the chloride channel (*CLCN7*). Candidate genes located in regions of suggestive or significant linkage for BMD regulation identified by genome-wide scans have also been investigated for their association with osteoporosis-related phenotypes. The most widely studied candidate genes that have been implicated in the regulation of BMD and other osteoporosis-related phenotypes are discussed in more detail in this section.

Vitamin D receptor

Vitamin D has important effects on bone and calcium metabolism through interaction with its nuclear receptor: the vitamin D receptor encoded by the *VDR* gene.

The *VDR* was the first candidate gene to be studied in relation to osteoporosis. Several *VDR* polymorphisms have now been studied in relation to BMD and other bone-related phenotypes, such as bone loss, osteocalcin levels, and osteoporotic fracture [44,45]. The most widely studied polymorphisms are *BsmI* and *ApaI*, located in intron 8, and *TaqI*, which is a conservative T→C change located in exon 9. Following the first report of an association between these polymorphisms and BMD by Morrison and colleagues [44], a large number of studies were performed with inconsistent results.

The majority of these studies have been summarized in two recent meta-analyses performed by Gong and colleagues [46] and Thakkinstian and colleagues [47]. The first study analyzed the outcomes of 75 studies published between 1994 and 1998. It concluded that there is a significant association between *VDR* polymorphisms and BMD, although the effect is small, and positive association with *VDR* polymorphisms was more common in studies that included premenopausal women rather than postmenopausal women. Furthermore, the investigators suggested that the association may have been missed in some studies because of small sample size and the effect of other confounding factors. Consistent with this suggestion, the relationship between *VDR* polymorphisms and BMD has been reported to be modified by environmental factors such as calcium and vitamin D intake [48]. The second meta-analysis analyzed studies published between 1994 and 2001 and included those that only genotyped the *BsmI* polymorphism in women [47]. The study found evidence for lower lumbar spine BMD (2.4%) in "*BsmI*" BB compared with Bb/bb genotypes, but no evidence for an association with femoral neck BMD. Fracture has also been studied by various investigators in relation to the *BsmI VDR* polymorphism, but results were inconsistent [45,49,50].

Functional studies performed to assess the effect of the *BsmI, ApaI*, and *TaqI* polymorphisms on *VDR* function or gene transcription have yielded inconsistent results. One study reported an evidence of haplotype-specific differences in gene transcription using reporter gene constructs prepared from the 3′ region of the *VDR* gene [44]. Other studies have shown no differences in allele-specific transcription, mRNA stability, or ligand binding [51] in relation to the polymorphisms in the 3′ region of the *VDR* gene, suggesting that these polymorphisms might be in linkage disequilibrium with other functional polymorphisms located in the *VDR* gene.

A functional polymorphism (recognized by the *FokI* restriction enzyme) in exon 2 of the *VDR* gene has been identified; it introduces an alternative translational start site, resulting in a shorter isoform of the *VDR* gene [52]. Studies of the association between the *FokI* polymorphism and BMD yielded inconsistent results [52], and studies of the effect of this polymorphism on the *VDR* function or transcription level were inconclusive [53]. Further studies are required to elucidate the effects of this polymorphism.

Another potentially functional polymorphism has been described in the *VDR* promoter at a binding site for the transcription factor Cdx-2 and has been found to be associated with BMD in Japanese subjects [54]. It was also reported to influence DNA protein binding and to modulate gene expression in reporter assays [54].

Recently, a large-scale study of the *VDR* gene in relation to the osteoporosis-related phenotype has been reported by Fang and colleagues [55]. Participants in the Rotterdam study (N = 6148) were genotyped for 15 haplotype-tagging SNPs selected after construction of linkage disequilibrium blocks across the *VDR* gene. The authors identified haplotype alleles in the promoter and the 3′ untranslated region (UTR) that were associated with increased risk for fracture. They observed a 48% increase in fracture risk in the subgroup of individuals (16%) who had risk genotypes at both regions, and this was independent of BMD. Functional analysis of *VDR* variants showed lower expression of a reporter construct with promoter risk haplotype and lower mRNA level of *VDR* expression constructs carrying 3′-UTR risk haplotype associated with increased degradation of *VDR* mRNA. Therefore, carriers of risk haplotypes at both promoter and 3′ UTR have lower *VDR* mRNA levels, attributed to the combined effect of decreased transcription and increased degradation of *VDR* mRNA. The authors suggested that lower *VDR* levels could affect the vitamin D signaling efficiency, which might contribute to the increased fracture risk, although the mechanism by which these variants predispose to fracture is unclear. Because the observed increase in fracture risk associated with risk haplotypes was independent of BMD, a possible effect on bone geometry may explain the observed increase in fracture risk. However, further studies will be required to confirm this hypothesis.

Collagen type I alpha 1

Collagen is the main structural protein of bone and is encoded by two separate genes: the *COLIA1* gene, which encodes the alpha 1 chain of type I collagen, and the *COLIA2* gene, which encodes the alpha 2 chain of type 1 collagen. Both genes are important functional candidate genes for the genetic regulation of bone mass and osteoporosis, because mutations in these genes account for the vast majority of osteogenesis imperfecta cases [56]. Although mutations affecting the coding region of the type I collagen genes have been excluded as a common cause of osteoporosis [57], attention has focused on the possibility that more subtle polymorphisms affecting the regulatory region of the collagen genes might predispose to osteoporosis. Most attention has been focused on a common polymorphism (G→T) located in intron 1 of the *COLIA1* gene, which was found to alter an Sp1 transcription binding site [58]. Grant and colleagues [58] reported a strong association between this polymorphism and osteoporosis. Following this report, extensive studies performed on this polymorphism have shown an association with BMD [58,59] and other osteoporosis-related phenotypes, such as fracture risk [58,59], bone loss [60,61], bone geometry [62], bone mineralization [63], and bone quality [64]. However, some studies reported no association between the *COLIA1* Sp1 polymorphism and BMD or fracture. Three meta-analyses of published studies investigating the Sp1 polymorphism have been performed and have concluded that the "T" allele of this polymorphism is associated with reduced BMD at lumbar spine and femoral neck and with increased risk for vertebral fractures [64–66]. Similar conclusions were reported in the large multicenter genetic markers for osteoporosis (GENOMOS) study [67], where the Sp1 polymorphism was genotyped in 20,786 individuals from several centers across Europe, and significant associations with BMD and incident vertebral fractures were found. Interestingly, this study showed a recessive effect of the Sp1 polymorphism on BMD, contrasting with a codominant effect reported in previous studies, although the association with vertebral fracture was mediated by a codominant effect as previously reported.

Functional studies of the *COLIA1* Sp1 polymorphism have shown evidence that the "T" allele is associated with increased binding affinity for Sp1 protein, threefold increase in the primary RNA transcripts, and increased production of type I alpha protein [64]. Furthermore, biomechanical testing of bone samples showed reduced bone strength and a slight reduction in mineralization of bone from samples with the "T" allele [63].

Recently, two polymorphisms (-1997G/T and -1663delT) have been described in the promoter of *COLIA1* gene that are in linkage disequilibrium with the Sp1 polymorphism and were found to be associated with BMD in some [68] but not other studies [69–71]. Functional analysis using reporter assays showed that these polymorphisms may affect *COLIA1* transcription [72].

More recently, a large study that included the promoter and the Sp1 polymorphism showed a consistent association with haplotypes that had opposing effects on both hip and spine BMD. These were haplotype 2 (-1997G/-1663DelT/Sp1"T"), which was significantly associated with low BMD, and haplotype 3 (-1997T/-1663InsT/Sp1"G"), which was significantly associated with high BMD [73]. These findings suggest that the association with Sp1 polymorphism previously reported by various studies may actually be driven by an extended haplotype spanning the promoter and intron 1 of *COLIA1* gene. The inconsistent results reported for the Sp1 polymorphism may be attributed to differences in the pattern of linkage disequilibrium among different populations.

Estrogen receptor alpha

Given that estrogen deficiency following the menopause is a major risk factor for osteoporosis, the estrogen receptor alpha encoded by the *ESR1* gene represents an important candidate gene for the genetic control of osteoporosis. Three main polymorphisms of the *ESR1* gene have been investigated: a thymine-adenine (TA) repeat polymorphism in the promoter region and two SNPs located in the first intron and defined by the restriction enzymes *PvuII* and *XbaI*.

The TA repeat polymorphism was first reported to be associated with BMD by Sano and colleagues [74], and the intron 1 *PvuII* and *XbaI* polymorphisms were first shown to be associated with BMD in a different study of Japanese subjects [75]. Subsequently, these polymorphisms have been investigated in relation to BMD [75–77] and other osteoporosis-related phenotypes [78,79], with mixed results. Ioannidis and colleagues [80] analyzed 22 studies published between 1996 and 2001 in a meta-analysis that showed evidence for an association between *XbaI* polymorphism and both BMD and fracture. They found that "XX" homozygotes were associated with higher BMD values and reduced risk for fractures compared with other genotype groups. A more recent and large-scale prospective meta-analysis of data from 18,917 individuals from the GENOMOS study showed that "XX" homozygotes were associated with reduced fracture risk, confirming the observation from the first meta-analysis [81]. However, no association with BMD was observed in this study, suggesting that *ESR1* polymorphisms might influence fracture risk by mechanisms that are independent of BMD, such as bone quality. Consistent with this finding, a recent study has shown a significant association of *ESR1* polymorphisms with ultrasound properties of bone and rates of postmenopausal bone loss in a large cohort of approximately 3000 women [82].

The data assembled so far indicate that allelic variation at the *ESR1* gene contributes to the genetic regulation of osteoporosis. Although there is evidence from reporter gene assays to suggest that the *PvuII* polymorphism creates a functional binding site for the transcription factor B-Myb [83], the impact of this polymorphism on *ESR1* transcription has not been determined. Further studies are required to elucidate the mechanisms by which *ESR1* alleles regulate bone phenotypes.

Transforming growth factor beta 1

The transforming growth factor beta 1 (*TGFβ1*) gene has been extensively studied as a potential regulator of susceptibility to osteoporosis, in part because it is particularly abundant in bone and has been shown to have effects on both osteoblast and osteoclast function in vitro [84]. One of the earliest studies was that of Langdahl and colleagues [85], who identified a polymorphism within intron 4 of the *TGFβ1* that was associated with severe osteoporosis. Subsequent work by the same group evaluated the relationship between several polymorphisms in *TGFβ1* and osteoporosis in a case control study and identified an association between a polymorphism located in the fifth intron and BMD [86]. Other research has focused on polymorphisms in the promoter and first exon of *TGFβ1* in relation to BMD [87–89]. A protein-coding polymorphism causing a leucine-to-proline substitution in the signal peptide region of *TGFβ1* has been found to be associated with BMD and with circulating *TGFβ1* in some populations [87,89], although the mechanism by which this polymorphism regulates BMD is unclear. Many studies of *TGFβ1* alleles in relation to BMD and other osteoporosis phenotypes have been performed, but most have been of limited sample size. Consequently, somewhat conflicting results have been reported. Definitive evidence that genetic variation in *TGFβ1* can regulate bone mass in humans comes from the observation that Camurati-Engelmann disease (a rare bone dysplasia characterized by osteosclerosis affecting the diaphysis of long bones) is caused by mutations in *TGFβ1* [90,91]. These mutations activate *TGFβ1* signaling by inhibiting binding of the mature *TGFβ1* peptide to the inhibitory latency-associated peptide [92].

Lipoprotein receptor–related protein 5

Various mutations in the lipoprotein receptor–related protein 5 (*LRP5*) gene were recently found to be responsible for two rare bone disorders: osteoporosis-pseudoglioma syndrome (OPS, a disorder characterized by juvenile onset osteoporosis and visual loss) and autosomal dominant inheritance of high bone mass (HBM) [93–95]. Inactivating mutations of *LRP5* are responsible for OPS, whereas gain-of-function mutations are responsible for the HBM syndrome. The *LRP5* gene encodes a transmembrane receptor, which is involved in *Wnt* signaling [95], and several polymorphisms of the *LRP5* gene have now been investigated in relation to BMD. Ferrari and colleagues [96] analyzed several polymorphisms of the *LRP5* gene in relation to BMD and identified significant association between G2047A polymorphism and lumbar spine BMD, but the association was most significant in men. However, subsequent studies have reported association between BMD and various haplotypes defined by polymorphisms in the *LRP5* in both men and women [97,98].

Current evidence suggests that the *LRP5* pathway regulates bone mass mainly by affecting bone formation. This is reflected by the observation that individuals with activating mutations have increased biochemical markers of bone formation, but no disturbance in bone resorption [95]. Consistent with this suggestion, heterozygous *LRP5* knockout mice have decreased trabecular bone volume density [99], and mice with HBM *LRP5* G171V mutation have increased bone cross-sectional area and thickness [100]. Functional analysis of the HBM-associated mutations of *LRP5* has shown that they probably cause activation of beta-catenin signaling by inhibiting interactions between *LRP5* and the inhibitor of *Wnt* signaling *Dkk1*. An initial study by Boyden and colleagues [95] showed that the G171V mutation did not result in constitutive activation of *LRP5* signaling in vitro but that it impaired *Dkk1*-mediated inhibition of *Wnt*-stimulated *LRP5* signaling. Another study reached the same conclusion in showing that several HBM-associated mutants (G171V, G171R, A214T, A214V, A242T, T253I, and D111Y) were resistant to *Dkk1* inhibition compared with wild type *LRP5* and had lower affinity for *Dkk1* binding [101]. Although the mechanisms by which rare *LRP5* mutations affect bone turnover appear to be reasonably well worked out, further studies are required to define the mechanism by which the more subtle polymorphisms in *LRP5* affect bone mass.

Core-binding factor A 1

The core-binding factor A 1 (*CBFA1*) gene (also known as *RUNX2*) plays an essential role in regulating osteoblast differentiation. Mice that are deficient in this transcription factor have complete absence of bone [102,103], whereas mice with haploinsufficiency of *CBFA1* phenocopy the human syndrome of cleidocranial dysplasia (CCD), a skeletal disorder characterized by short stature, hypoplasia or aplasia of the clavicles, patent fontanelles, supernumerary teeth, and other defects in skeletal patterning and growth [103]. The human syndrome of CCD is caused by various missense, nonsense, and frameshift mutations of *CBFA1* [104]. Various polymorphisms have been identified in *CBFA1*, and some of these have been associated with bone mass in population-based studies [105–107]. The best functional candidate polymorphisms lie within the *CBFA1* promoter or within polyalanine and polyglutamine repeats in exon 1 [105]. The polyalanine and polyglutamine repeats are of special interest, because they lie within one of the transactivation domains of *CBFA1*. Various polymorphic variations have been identified in this region, including an *18bp* deletion that results in a polyalanine repeat of 11 residues (11 ala) compared with the more common repeat of 17 residues (17 ala). Various rare length variants within the polyglutamine repeat have also been identified, resulting in stretches of between 15 and 30 repeats. The strongest association with BMD has been observed with an anonymous polymorphism in the ala repeat region [106,107]. However, it is believed that this may be due to linkage disequilibrium with polymorphisms in the promoter, which have been shown to affect *CBFA1* transcription in reporter assays [105]. It is currently unclear whether the length variants in the polyalanine and polyglutamine tracts have functional importance, but this is an area of ongoing investigation.

Tumor necrosis factor receptor superfamily 1B

The tumor necrosis factor receptor superfamily 1B (*TNFRSF1B*; also known as *TNFR2*) mediates the effects of TNF, which have an important role in regulating bone turnover. Specifically, TNF-α–induced activation of the *TNFRSF1B* receptor has been found to suppress osteoclastogenesis in vitro, in contrast with its effects on the *TNFRSF1A* receptor, which result in enhanced osteoclastogenesis [108]. The *TNFRSF1B* gene is located on the chromosome 1p36 region that was found to be linked to BMD in three independent studies, rendering it both a positional and functional candidate for the regulation of BMD [20,109,110]. Polymorphisms in the 3′ UTR of *TNFRSF1B* have been reported to be associated with spine BMD in a small population based study of an American population [111]. However, a larger study in Scottish women showed an association with femoral neck but not lumbar spine BMD [112], consistent with the linkage findings identified by genome-wide linkage scan [20]. Because these polymorphisms are located in the 3′ UTR, it has been postulated that they may influence *TNFRSF1B* mRNA level by affecting the mRNA structure and stability.

Chloride channel 7 and osteoclast-specific proton pump

Mutations in genes encoding chloride channel 7 (*CLCN7*) and osteoclast-specific proton pump (*TCIRG1*) have been found to cause some forms of osteopetrosis [113], a disease characterized by increased BMD due to impaired osteoclast function. Both genes are highly expressed in osteoclast and play a significant role in acidification of the lacunae during bone resorption. Polymorphisms in the *CLCN7* and *TCIRG1* have been reported to be associated with BMD [114,115]; however, further studies in different populations will be required to confirm these findings.

Other candidate genes

Polymorphisms of many other candidate genes have been studied in relation to BMD and other osteoporosis-related phenotypes (reviewed by Liu and colleagues [116]). Constraints of space do not permit full discussion of these genes, which in general have been investigated in populations with a limited sample size. Further studies will be required to confirm their candidacy as genetic regulators of bone mass.

Summary

Over the past 10 years, many advances have been made in understanding the mechanisms by which genetic factors regulate susceptibility to osteoporosis. It has become clear from studies in man and experimental animals that different genes regulate BMD at different skeletal sites and in men and women. Linkage studies have identified several chromosomal regions that regulate BMD, but only a few causative genes have been discovered so far using this approach. In contrast, significant advances have been made in identifying the genes that cause monogenic bone diseases, and polymorphic variation in some of these genes has been found to contribute to the genetic regulation of BMD in the normal population. Other genes that have been investigated as possible candidates for susceptibility to osteoporosis because of their role in bone biology, such as vitamin D, have yielded mixed results. Many candidate gene association studies have been underpowered, and meta-analysis has been used to try to confirm or refute potential associations and gain a better estimate of their true effect size in the population. Most of the genetic variants that confer susceptibility to osteoporosis remain to be discovered. It is likely that new techniques such as whole-genome association will provide new insights into the genetic determinants of osteoporosis and will help to identify genes of modest effect size. From a clinical standpoint, genetic variants that are found to predispose to osteoporosis will advance our understanding of the pathophysiology of the disease. They could be developed as diagnostic genetic tests or form molecular targets for design of new drugs for the prevention and treatment of osteoporosis and other bone diseases.

References

[1] Cummings SR, Nevitt MC, Browner WS, et al. Risk factors for hip fracture in white women. Study of Osteoporotic Fractures Research Group. N Engl J Med 1995;332(12): 767–73.

[2] Soroko SB, Barret-Connor E, Edelstein SL, et al. Family history of osteoporosis and bone mineral density at the axial skeleton: the Rancho Bernardo study. J Bone Miner Res 1994;9: 761–9.

[3] Pocock NA, Eisman JA, Hopper JL, et al. Genetic determinants of bone mass in adults: a twin study. J Clin Invest 1987;80:706–10.

[4] Slemenda CW, Christian JC, Williams CJ, et al. Genetic determinants of bone mass in adult women: a reevaluation of the twin model and the potential importance of gene interaction on heritability estimates. J Bone Miner Res 1991;6:561–7.

[5] Gueguen R, Jouanny P, Guillemin F, et al. Segregation analysis and variance components analysis of bone mineral density in healthy families. J Bone Miner Res 1995;12:2017–22.

[6] Krall EA, Dawson-Hughes B. Heritable and life-style determinants of bone mineral density. J Bone Miner Res 1993;8:1–9.

[7] Torgerson DJ, Campbell MK, Thomas RE, et al. Prediction of perimenopausal fractures by bone mineral density and other risk factors. J Bone Miner Res 1996;11(2):293–7.

[8] Arden NK, Baker J, Hogg C, et al. The heritability of bone mineral density, ultrasound of the calcaneus and hip axis length: a study of postmenopausal twins. J Bone Miner Res 1996; 11:530–4.

[9] Arden NK, Spector TD. Genetic influences on muscle strength, lean body mass, and bone mineral density: a twin study. J Bone Miner Res 1997;12(12):2076–81.

[10] Hunter D, De Lange M, Snieder H, et al. Genetic contribution to bone metabolism, calcium excretion, and vitamin D and parathyroid hormone regulation. J Bone Miner Res 2001; 16(2):371–8.

[11] Kaprio J, Rimpela A, Winter T, et al. Common genetic influences on BMI and age at menarche. Hum Biol 1995;67(5):739–53.

[12] Kannus P, Palvanen M, Kaprio J, et al. Genetic factors and osteoporotic fractures in elderly people: prospective 25 year follow up of a nationwide cohort of elderly Finnish twins. BMJ 1999;319(7221):1334–7.

[13] Deng HW, Chen WM, Recker S, et al. Genetic determination of Colles' fracture and differential bone mass in women with and without Colles' fracture. J Bone Miner Res 2000;15(7): 1243–52.

[14] Andrew T, Antioniades L, Scurrah KJ, et al. Risk of wrist fracture in women is heritable and is influenced by genes that are largely independent of those influencing BMD. J Bone Miner Res 2005;20(1):67–74.

[15] Michaelsson K, Melhus H, Ferm H, et al. Genetic liability to fractures in the elderly. Arch Intern Med 2005;165(16):1825–30.

[16] Nyholt DR. All LODs are not created equal. Am J Hum Genet 2000;67(2):282–8.

[17] Sawcer SJ, Maranian M, Singlehurst S, et al. Enhancing linkage analysis of complex disorders: an evaluation of high-density genotyping. Hum Mol Genet 2004;13(17):1943–9.

[18] Gong Y, Vikkula M, Boon L, et al. Osteoporosis pseudoglioma syndrome, a disorder affecting skeletal strength and vision, is assigned to chromosome region 11q12-13. Am J Hum Genet 1996;59(1):146–51.

[19] Johnson ML, Gong G, Kimberling W, et al. Linkage of a gene causing high bone mass to human chromosome 11 (11q12-13). Am J Hum Genet 1997;60:1326–32.

[20] Devoto M, Shimoya K, Caminis J, et al. First-stage autosomal genome screen in extended pedigrees suggests genes predisposing to low bone mineral density on chromosomes 1p, 2p and 4q. Eur J Hum Genet 1998;6:151–7.

[21] Almasy L, Blangero J. Multipoint quantitative-trait linkage analysis in general pedigrees. Am J Hum Genet 1998;62(5):1198–211.

[22] Lee YH, Rho YH, Choi SJ, et al. Meta-analysis of genome-wide linkage studies for bone mineral density. J Hum Genet 2006;51(5):480–6.

[23] Koller DL, Liu G, Econs MJ, et al. Genome screen for quantitative trait loci underlying normal variation in femoral structure. J Bone Miner Res 2001;16(6):985–91.

[24] Wilson SG, Reed PW, Andrew T, et al. A genome-screen of a large twin cohort reveals linkage for quantitative ultrasound of the calcaneus to 2q33-37 and 4q12-21. J Bone Miner Res 2004;19(2):270–7.

[25] Peacock M, Koller DL, Lai D, et al. Sex-specific quantitative trait loci contribute to normal variation in bone structure at the proximal femur in men. Bone 2005;37(4):467–73.

[26] Ralston SH, Galwey N, MacKay I, et al. Loci for regulation of bone mineral density in men and women identified by genome wide linkage scan: the FAMOS study. Hum Mol Genet 2005;14(7):943–51.

[27] Styrkarsdottir U, Cazier JB, Kong A, et al. Linkage of osteoporosis to chromosome 20p12 and association to BMP2. PLoS Biol 2003;1(3):e69.

[28] Klein RF, Mitchell SR, Phillips TJ, et al. Quantitative trait loci affecting peak bone mineral density in mice. J Bone Miner Res 1998;13(11):1648–56.

[29] Shimizu M, Higuchi K, Bennett B, et al. Identification of peak bone mass QTL in a spontaneously osteoporotic mouse strain. Mamm Genome 1999;10:81–7.

[30] Beamer WG, Shultz KL, Churchill GA, et al. Quantitative trait loci for bone density in C57BL/6J and CAST/EiJ inbred mice. Mamm Genome 1999;10(11):1043–9.

[31] Benes H, Weinstein RS, Zheng W, et al. Chromosomal mapping of osteopenia-associated quantitative trait loci using closely related mouse strains. J Bone Miner Res 2000;15(4): 626–33.

[32] Klein RF, Turner RJ, Skinner LD, et al. Mapping quantitative trait loci that influence femoral cross-sectional area in mice. J Bone Miner Res 2002;17(10):1752–60.

[33] Bouxsein ML, Uchiyama T, Rosen CJ, et al. Mapping quantitative trait loci for vertebral trabecular bone volume fraction and microarchitecture in mice. J Bone Miner Res 2004; 19(4):587–99.

[34] Volkman SK, Galecki AT, Burke DT, et al. Quantitative trait loci that modulate femoral mechanical properties in a genetically heterogeneous mouse population. J Bone Miner Res 2004;19(9):1497–505.

[35] Orwoll ES, Belknap JK, Klein RF. Gender specificity in the genetic determinants of peak bone mass. J Bone Miner Res 2001;16(11):1962–71.

[36] Turner CH, Sun Q, Schriefer J, et al. Congenic mice reveal sex-specific genetic regulation of femoral structure and strength. Calcif Tissue Int 2003;73(3):297–303.

[37] Beamer WG, Shultz KL, Donahue LR, et al. Quantitative trait loci for femoral and lumbar vertebral bone mineral density in C57BL/6J and C3H/HeJ inbred strains of mice. J Bone Miner Res 2001;16(7):1195–206.

[38] Masinde GL, Li X, Gu W, et al. Quantitative trait loci for bone density in mice: the genes determining total skeletal density and femur density show little overlap in F2 mice. Calcif Tissue Int 2002;71(5):421–8.

[39] Klein OF, Carlos AS, Vartanian KA, et al. Confirmation and fine mapping of chromosomal regions influencing peak bone mass in mice. J Bone Miner Res 2001;16(11): 1953–61.

[40] Klein RF, Allard J, Avnur Z, et al. Regulation of bone mass in mice by the lipoxygenase gene Alox15. Science 2004;303(5655):229–32.

[41] Urano T, Shiraki M, Fujita M, et al. Association of a single nucleotide polymorphism in the lipoxygenase ALOX15 5′-flanking region (-5229G/A) with bone mineral density. J Bone Miner Metab 2005;23(3):226–30.

[42] Parsons CA, Mroczkowski HJ, McGuigan FE, et al. Interspecies synteny mapping identifies a quantitative trait locus for bone mineral density on human chromosome Xp22. Hum Mol Genet 2005;14(21):3141–8.

[43] Cardon LR, Abecasis GR. Using haplotype blocks to map human complex trait loci. Trends Genet 2003;19(3):135–40.

[44] Morrison NA, Qi JC, Tokita A, et al. Prediction of bone density from vitamin D receptor alleles. Nature 1994;367:284–7.

[45] Uitterlinden AG, Weel AE, Burger H, et al. Interaction between the vitamin D receptor gene and collagen type I alpha 1 gene in susceptibility for fracture. J Bone Miner Res 2001;16(2):379–85.

[46] Gong G, Stern HS, Cheng SC, et al. The association of bone mineral density with vitamin D receptor gene polymorphisms. Osteoporos Int 1999;9(1):55–64.

[47] Thakkinstian A, D'Este C, Eisman J, et al. Meta-analysis of molecular association studies: vitamin D receptor gene polymorphisms and BMD as a case study. J Bone Miner Res 2004; 19(3):419–28.

[48] Graafmans WC, Lips P, Ooms ME, et al. The effect of vitamin D supplementation on the bone mineral density of the femoral neck is associated with vitamin D receptor genotype. J Bone Miner Res 1997;12(8):1241–5.

[49] Feskanich D, Hunter DJ, Willett WC, et al. Vitamin D receptor genotype and the risk of bone fractures in women. Epidemiology 1998;9(5):535–9.

[50] Ensrud KE, Stone K, Cauley JA, et al. Vitamin D receptor gene polymorphisms and the risk of fractures in older women. For the Study of Osteoporotic Fractures Research Group. J Bone Miner Res 1999;14(10):1637–45.

[51] Gross C, Musiol IM, Eccleshall TR, et al. Vitamin D receptor gene polymorphisms: analysis of ligand binding and hormone responsiveness in cultured skin fibroblasts. Biochem Biophys Res Commun 1998;242(3):467–73.

[52] Arai H, Miyamoto K-I, Taketani Y, et al. A vitamin D receptor gene polymorphism in the translation initiation codon: effect on protein activity and relation to bone mineral density in Japanese women. J Bone Miner Res 1997;12:915–21.

[53] Gross C, Krishnan AV, Malloy PJ, et al. The vitamin D receptor gene start codon polymorphism: a functional analysis of FokI variants. J Bone Miner Res 1998;13(11): 1691–9.

[54] Arai H, Miyamoto KI, Yoshida M, et al. The polymorphism in the caudal-related homeo-domain protein Cdx-2 binding element in the human vitamin D receptor gene. J Bone Miner Res 2001;16(7):1256–64.

[55] Fang Y, van Meurs JB, d'Alesio A, et al. Promoter and 3′-untranslated-region haplotypes in the vitamin D receptor gene predispose to osteoporotic fracture: the Rotterdam study. Am J Hum Genet 2005;77(5):807–23.

[56] Rowe DW. Osteogenesis imperfecta. In: Heersche JNM, Kanis JA, editors. Bone and mineral research. Amsterdam: Elsevier; 1991. p. 209–41.

[57] Spotila LD, Colige A, Sereda L, et al. Mutation analysis of coding sequences for type 1 procollagen in individuals with low bone density. J Bone Miner Res 1994;9:923–32.

[58] Grant SFA, Reid DM, Blake G, et al. Reduced bone density and osteoporosis associated with a polymorphic Sp1 site in the collagen type I alpha 1 gene. Nat Genet 1996;14:203–5.

[59] Uitterlinden AG, Burger H, Huang Q, et al. Relation of alleles of the collagen type I a 1 gene to bone density and risk of osteoporotic fractures in postmenopausal women. N Engl J Med 1998;338:1016–22.

[60] MacDonald HM, McGuigan FA, New SA, et al. COL1A1 Sp1 polymorphism predicts perimenopausal and early postmenopausal spinal bone loss. J Bone Miner Res 2001; 16(9):1634–41.

[61] Harris SS, Patel MS, Cole DE, et al. Associations of the collagen type I alpha 1 Sp1 polymorphism with five-year rates of bone loss in older adults. Calcif Tissue Int 2000;66(4): 268–71.

[62] Qureshi AM, McGuigan FEA, Seymour DG, et al. Association between COL1A1 Sp1 alleles and femoral neck geometry. Calcif Tissue Int 2001;69(2):67–72.

[63] Stewart TL, Roschger P, Misof BM, et al. Association of COL1A1 Sp1 alleles with defective bone nodule formation in vitro and abnormal bone mineralization in vivo. Calcif Tissue Int 2005;77(2):113–8.

[64] Mann V, Hobson EE, Li B, et al. A COL1A1 Sp1 binding site polymorphism predisposes to osteoporotic fracture by affecting bone density and quality. J Clin Invest 2001;107(7): 899–907.

[65] Mann V, Ralston SH. Meta-analysis of COL1A1 Sp1 polymorphism in relation to bone mineral density and osteoporotic fracture. Bone 2003;32(6):711–7.

[66] Efstathiadou Z, Tsatsoulis A, Ioannidis JP. Association of collagen I alpha 1 Sp1 polymorphism with the risk of prevalent fractures: a meta-analysis. J Bone Miner Res 2001;16(9): 1586–92.

[67] Ralston SH, Uitterlinden AG, Brandi ML, et al. Large-scale evidence for the effect of the COL1A1 Sp1 polymorphism on osteoporosis outcomes: the GENOMOS study. PLoS Med 2006;3(4):e90.

[68] Garcia-Giralt N, Nogues X, Enjuanes A, et al. Two new single nucleotide polymorphisms in the COL1A1 upstream regulatory region and their relationship with bone mineral density. J Bone Miner Res 2002;17(3):384–93.

[69] Zhang YY, Lei SF, Mo XY, et al. The -1997 G/T polymorphism in the COL1A1 upstream regulatory region is associated with hip bone mineral density (BMD) in Chinese nuclear families. Calcif Tissue Int 2005;76(2):107–12.

[70] Yamada Y, Ando F, Niino N, et al. Association of a -1997G→T polymorphism of the collagen I alpha 1 gene with bone mineral density in postmenopausal Japanese women. Hum Biol 2005;77(1):27–36.

[71] Liu PY, Lu Y, Long JR, et al. Common variants at the PCOL2 and Sp1 binding sites of the COL1A1 gene and their interactive effect influence bone mineral density in Caucasians. J Med Genet 2004;41(10):752–7.

[72] Garcia-Giralt N, Enjuanes A, Bustamante M, et al. In vitro functional assay of alleles and haplotypes of two COL1A1-promoter SNPs. Bone 2005;36(5):902–8.

[73] Stewart TL, Jin H, McGuigan FE, et al. Haplotypes defined by promoter and intron 1 polymorphisms of the COLIA1 gene regulate bone mineral density in women. J Clin Endocrinol Metab 2006;91(9):3575–83.

[74] Sano M, Inoue S, Hosoi T, et al. Association of estrogen receptor dinucleotide repeat polymorphism with osteoporosis. Biochem Biophys Res Commun 1995;217(1):378–83.

[75] Kobayashi S, Inoue S, Hosoi T, et al. Association of bone mineral density with polymorphisms of the estrogen receptor gene in post-menopausal women. J Bone Miner Res 1996;11:306–11.

[76] Willing M, Sowers M, Aron D, et al. Bone mineral density and its change in white women: estrogen and vitamin D receptor genotypes and their interaction. J Bone Miner Res 1998; 13(4):695–705.

[77] Albagha OM, McGuigan FE, Reid DM, et al. Estrogen receptor alpha gene polymorphisms and bone mineral density: haplotype analysis in women from the United Kingdom. J Bone Miner Res 2001;16(1):128–34.

[78] Salmen T, Heikkinen AM, Mahonen A, et al. Early postmenopausal bone loss is associated with PvuII estrogen receptor gene polymorphism in Finnish women: effect of hormone replacement therapy. J Bone Miner Res 2000;15(2):315–21.

[79] van Meurs JB, Schuit SC, Weel AE, et al. Association of 5′ estrogen receptor alpha gene polymorphisms with bone mineral density, vertebral bone area and fracture risk. Hum Mol Genet 2003;12(14):1745–54.

[80] Ioannidis JP, Stavrou I, Trikalinos TA, et al. Association of polymorphisms of the estrogen receptor alpha gene with bone mineral density and fracture risk in women: a meta-analysis. J Bone Miner Res 2002;17(11):2048–60.

[81] Ioannidis JP, Ralston SH, Bennett ST, et al. Differential genetic effects of ESR1 gene polymorphisms on osteoporosis outcomes. JAMA 2004;292(17):2105–14.

[82] Albagha OM, Pettersson U, Stewart A, et al. Association of oestrogen receptor alpha gene polymorphisms with postmenopausal bone loss, bone mass, and quantitative ultrasound properties of bone. J Med Genet 2005;42(3):240–6.

[83] Herrington DM, Howard TD, Brosnihan KB, et al. Common estrogen receptor polymorphism augments effects of hormone replacement therapy on E-selectin but not C-reactive protein. Circulation 2002;105(16):1879–82.

[84] Massague J, Chen YG. Controlling TGF-beta signaling. Genes Dev 2000;14(6):627–44.

[85] Langdahl BL, Knudsen JY, Jensen HK, et al. A sequence variation: 713-8delC in the transforming growth factor–beta 1 gene has higher prevalence in osteoporotic women than in normal women and is associated with very low bone mass in osteoporotic women and increased bone turnover in both osteoporotic and normal women. Bone 1997;20(3):289–94.

[86] Langdahl BL, Carstens M, Stenkjaer L, et al. Polymorphisms in the transforming growth factor beta 1 gene and osteoporosis. Bone 2003;32(3):297–310.

[87] Yamada Y, Hosoi T, Makimoto F, et al. Transforming growth factor beta–1 gene polymorphism and bone mineral density in Japanese adolescents. Am J Med 1999;106(4):477–9.

[88] Hinke V, Seck T, Clanget C, et al. Association of transforming growth factor–beta1 (TGF-beta1) T29 → C gene polymorphism with bone mineral density (BMD), changes in BMD, and serum concentrations of TGF-beta1 in a population-based sample of postmenopausal German women. Calcif Tissue Int 2001;69(6):315–20.

[89] Yamada Y, Miyauchi A, Takagi Y, et al. Association of the C-509→T polymorphism, alone or in combination with the T869→C polymorphism, of the transforming growth

factor–beta1 gene with bone mineral density and genetic susceptibility to osteoporosis in Japanese women. J Mol Med 2001;79(2–3):149–56.

[90] Kinoshita A, Saito T, Tomita H, et al. Domain-specific mutations in TGFB1 result in Camurati-Engelmann disease. Nat Genet 2000;26(1):19–20.

[91] Janssens K, Gershoni-Baruch R, Guanabens N, et al. Mutations in the gene encoding the latency-associated peptide of TGF–beta 1 cause Camurati-Engelmann disease. Nat Genet 2000;26(3):273–5.

[92] Janssens K, ten Dijke P, Ralston SH, et al. Transforming growth factor–beta 1 mutations in Camurati-Engelmann disease lead to increased signaling by altering either activation or secretion of the mutant protein. J Biol Chem 2003;278(9):7718–24.

[93] Gong Y, Slee RB, Fukai N, et al. LDL receptor–related protein 5 (LRP5) affects bone accrual and eye development. Cell 2001;107(4):513–23.

[94] Little RD, Carulli JP, Del Mastro RG, et al. A mutation in the LDL receptor–related protein 5 gene results in the autosomal dominant high-bone-mass trait. Am J Hum Genet 2002; 70(1):11–9.

[95] Boyden LM, Mao J, Belsky J, et al. High bone density due to a mutation in LDL-receptor–related protein 5. N Engl J Med 2002;346(20):1513–21.

[96] Ferrari SL, Deutsch S, Choudhury U, et al. Polymorphisms in the low-density lipoprotein receptor–related protein 5 (LRP5) gene are associated with variation in vertebral bone mass, vertebral bone size, and stature in whites. Am J Hum Genet 2004;74(5):866–75.

[97] Koller DL, Ichikawa S, Johnson ML, et al. Contribution of the LRP5 gene to normal variation in peak BMD in women. J Bone Miner Res 2005;20(1):75–80.

[98] Ferrari SL, Deutsch S, Antonarakis SE. Pathogenic mutations and polymorphisms in the lipoprotein receptor–related protein 5 reveal a new biological pathway for the control of bone mass. Curr Opin Lipidol 2005;16(2):207–14.

[99] Holmen SL, Giambernardi TA, Zylstra CR, et al. Decreased BMD and limb deformities in mice carrying mutations in both Lrp5 and Lrp6. J Bone Miner Res 2004;19(12):2033–40.

[100] Akhter MP, Wells DJ, Short SJ, et al. Bone biomechanical properties in LRP5 mutant mice. Bone 2004;35(1):162–9.

[101] Ai M, Holmen SL, Van Hul W, et al. Reduced affinity to and inhibition by DKK1 form a common mechanism by which high bone mass–associated missense mutations in LRP5 affect canonical Wnt signaling. Mol Cell Biol 2005;25(12):4946–55.

[102] Komori T, Yagi H, Nomura S, et al. Targeted disruption of Cbfa1 results in a complete lack of bone formation owing to maturational arrest of osteoblasts. Cell 1997;89:755–64.

[103] Otto F, Thornell AP, Crompton T, et al. Cbfa1, a candidate gene for cleidocranial dysplasia syndrome, is essential for osteoblast differentiation and bone development. Cell 1997;89(5): 765–71.

[104] Quack I, Vonderstrass B, Stock M, et al. Mutation analysis of core binding factor A1 in patients with cleidocranial dysplasia. Am J Hum Genet 1999;65(5):1268–78.

[105] Doecke JD, Day CJ, Stephens AS, et al. Association of functionally different RUNX2 P2 promoter alleles with BMD. J Bone Miner Res 2006;21(2):265–73.

[106] Vaughan T, Reid DM, Morrison NA, et al. RUNX2 alleles associated with BMD in Scottish women; interaction of RUNX2 alleles with menopausal status and body mass index. Bone 2004;34(6):1029–36.

[107] Vaughan T, Pasco JA, Kotowicz MA, et al. Alleles of RUNX2/CBFA1 gene are associated with differences in bone mineral density and risk of fracture. J Bone Miner Res 2002;17(8): 1527–34.

[108] Abu-Amer Y, Erdmann J, Alexopoulou L, et al. Tumor necrosis factor receptors types 1 and 2 differentially regulate osteoclastogenesis. J Biol Chem 2000;275(35):27307–10.

[109] Devoto M, Specchia C, Li HH, et al. Variance component linkage analysis indicates a QTL for femoral neck bone mineral density on chromosome 1p36. Hum Mol Genet 2001;10(21): 2447–52.

[110] Wilson SG, Reed PW, Bansal A, et al. Comparison of genome screens for two independent cohorts provides replication of suggestive linkage of bone mineral density to 3p21 and 1p36. Am J Hum Genet 2003;72(1):144–55.

[111] Spotila LD, Rodriguez H, Koch M, et al. Association of a polymorphism in the TNFR2 gene with low bone mineral density. J Bone Miner Res 2000;15(7):1376–83.

[112] Albagha OM, Tasker PN, McGuigan FE, et al. Linkage disequilibrium between polymorphisms in the human TNFRSF1B gene and their association with bone mass in perimenopausal women. Hum Mol Genet 2002;11(19):2289–95.

[113] Balemans W, Van Wesenbeeck L, Van Hul W. A clinical and molecular overview of the human osteopetroses. Calcif Tissue Int 2005;77(5):263–74.

[114] Sobacchi C, Vezzoni P, Reid DM, et al. Association between a polymorphism affecting an AP1 binding site in the promoter of the TCIRG1 gene and bone mass in women. Calcif Tissue Int 2004;74(1):35–41.

[115] Pettersson U, Albagha OM, Mirolo M, et al. Polymorphisms of the CLCN7 gene are associated with BMD in women. J Bone Miner Res 2005;20(11):1960–7.

[116] Liu YZ, Liu YJ, Recker RR, et al. Molecular studies of identification of genes for osteoporosis: the 2002 update. J Endocrinol 2003;177(2):147–96.

[117] Niu T, Chen C, Cordell H, et al. A genome-wide scan for loci linked to forearm bone mineral density. Hum Genet 1999;104(3):226–33.

[118] Koller DL, Econs MJ, Morin PA, et al. Genome screen for QTLs contributing to normal variation in bone mineral density and osteoporosis. J Clin Endocrinol Metab 2000;85(9): 3116–20.

[119] Karasik D, Myers RH, Cupples LA, et al. Genome screen for quantitative trait loci contributing to normal variation in bone mineral density: the Framingham Study. J Bone Miner Res 2002;17(9):1718–27.

[120] Deng HW, Xu FH, Huang QY, et al. A whole-genome linkage scan suggests several genomic regions potentially containing quantitative trait loci for osteoporosis. J Clin Endocrinol Metab 2002;87(11):5151–9.

[121] Karasik D, Cupples LA, Hannan MT, et al. Age, gender, and body mass effects on quantitative trait loci for bone mineral density: the Framingham Study. Bone 2003;33(3):308–16.

[122] Kammerer CM, Schneider JL, Cole SA, et al. Quantitative trait loci on chromosomes 2p, 4p, and 13q influence bone mineral density of the forearm and hip in Mexican Americans. J Bone Miner Res 2003;18(12):2245–52.

[123] Shen H, Zhang YY, Long JR, et al. A genome-wide linkage scan for bone mineral density in an extended sample: evidence for linkage on 11q23 and Xq27. J Med Genet 2004;41(10): 743–51.

[124] Peacock M, Koller DL, Fishburn T, et al. Sex-specific and non–sex-specific quantitative trait loci contribute to normal variation in bone mineral density in men. J Clin Endocrinol Metab 2005;90(5):3060–6.

ELSEVIER
SAUNDERS

RHEUMATIC
DISEASE CLINICS
OF NORTH AMERICA

Rheum Dis Clin N Am 32 (2006) 681–689

Recommendations for Measurement of Bone Mineral Density and Identifying Persons to be Treated for Osteoporosis

Marc C. Hochberg, MD, MPH[a,b,*]

[a]Division of Rheumatology, Department of Medicine and Department
of Epidemiology and Preventive Medicine, University of Maryland School of Medicine,
10 South Pine Street, MSTF 8-34 Baltimore, MD 21201, USA
[b]Maryland Veterans Affairs Health Care System, 10 N. Greene Street,
Baltimore, MD 21201, USA

Osteoporosis has been defined as a systemic skeletal disorder that is characterized by compromised bone strength that predisposes to an increased risk for fracture [1]. Bone strength is determined by many factors, including bone mass and bone quality. Bone mass is estimated in clinical practice by the measurement of bone mineral density (BMD). Areal BMD, as measured by dual x-ray absorptiometry (DXA), represents an estimate of the quantity of mineral (grams of calcium) divided by the two-dimensional area of the bone. There is a strong nonlinear relationship between BMD and the risk for fracture; for every one standard deviation decrease below the age-adjusted mean for femoral neck BMD, the risk for hip fracture increases by a factor of greater than two [2]. The World Health Organization defined osteoporosis in white women as a BMD measured at the femoral neck of 2.5 or more standard deviations below the mean of young white women aged 20 to 29 years [3]. This definition has been generalized to nonwhite women and men with the proviso that normative data for young persons be sex-specific. In its most recently position statement, the International Society for Clinical Densitometry (ISCD) stated that "[o]steoporosis may be diagnosed in postmenopausal women and in men age 50 and older if the T-score of the lumbar spine, total hip or femoral neck is −2.5 or less" [4].

The most important osteoporotic fractures, from the standpoint of incidence and consequences, are vertebral and hip fractures [5–7]. Results of

* Division of Rheumatology, Department of Medicine and Department of Epidemiology
and Preventive Medicine, University of Maryland School of Medicine, 10 South Pine Street,
MSTF 8-34 Baltimore, MD 21201.
 E-mail address: mhochber@umaryland.edu

0889-857X/06/$ - see front matter © 2006 Elsevier Inc. All rights reserved.
doi:10.1016/j.rdc.2006.09.002
rheumatic.theclinics.com

randomized placebo-controlled clinical trials demonstrated that treatment of postmenopausal women who have prevalent vertebral fractures or low BMD (lumbar spine or femoral neck T-score of −2.0 or less) can reduce the risk for vertebral, nonvertebral, and hip fractures [8–10]. Similarly, treatment of men who had low BMD reduced the risk for vertebral fractures [11,12].

This article reviews recommendations and algorithms for identifying persons who should undergo measurement of BMD, and, if appropriate, treatment, to reduce their risk for fracture. The article does not cover treatment for the purpose of prevention of further bone loss in persons who do not have osteoporosis.

Who should have bone mineral density measured?

Morris and colleagues [13] performed a systematic review of MEDLINE and HealthSTAR from 1992 through 2002 to identify clinical practice guideline for screening for osteoporosis. Of 36 published clinical practice guidelines, they selected 17 for detailed review. Among 11 guidelines that considered postmenopausal women, 6 guidelines (53%) recommended universal screening at age 65 years and older; all guidelines endorsed screening of younger postmenopausal women who have risk factors for fracture, although there was no agreement of specific risk factors to be used. The most commonly cited risk factors were previous fracture, family history of osteoporosis or osteoporotic fracture, alcohol use, current smoking, and low body mass index. In a review of seven studies that examined BMD testing in patients who had fractures, the proportion that underwent BMD testing ranged from 1% to 32%, with a weighted mean of 8%.

Elliot-Gibson and colleagues [14] performed a systematic review of MEDLINE, HealthSTAR, CINAHL, EMBASE, Premedline, the Cochrane Register of Controlled Trials, and the Cochrane Database of Systematic Reviews from January 1994 through January 2003 to identify studies that reported on the clinical practice for the diagnosis and treatment of osteoporosis in patients who had experienced a fracture. The investigators reviewed 37 articles, 29 of which reported on rates of osteoporosis investigation, diagnosis, or treatment in patients who sustained fractures. Sixteen studies reported that BMD was measured by DXA in patients who had experienced a fracture. The proportion tested ranged from 0.5% to 32% in 14 of these studies, and it was 100% in the remaining 2 studies; the median proportion was 8%. The investigators concluded that investigation for osteoporosis in patients who had experienced a fracture was low, and that potential barriers to screening and diagnosis of osteoporosis included a lack of clarity concerning the clinical responsibility for osteoporosis diagnosis and care, time and cost of diagnosis, and concerns about polypharmacy, especially in an older population.

More recently, Lewiecki [15] also reviewed clinical practice guidelines for BMD testing and treatment of osteoporosis. He performed a systematic review of MEDLINE and the National Guideline Clearinghouse to identify clinical practice guidelines that were written in English; distributed widely in the United States; and published, updated, or endorsed since the year 2000. Seventy-eight clinical practice guidelines for BMD testing were identified; of these, there were 6 unique published guidelines (Box 1) [1,4,16–19]. The most widely recognized guidelines are those of the National Osteoporosis Foundation (NOF) [16]. The NOF recommends BMD testing in all postmenopausal white women aged 65 years and older, as well as in younger postmenopausal white women with one or more of the following risk factors: personal history of low-trauma clinical fracture after age 50 years, history of osteoporotic fracture in a first-degree relative, low body weight (127 pounds or less), or current smoking. These recommendations, although only written to apply directly to white women, have been expanded liberally for all women. The NOF is developing recommendations for BMD testing in men.

The American Association of Clinical Endocrinologists (AACE) also recommends that postmenopausal women aged 65 years and older should undergo BMD testing [17]. In addition, younger postmenopausal women with a history of a clinical fracture that was not caused by major trauma (eg, motor vehicle accident), as well as those with other risk factors for fracture, should undergo BMD testing. These other risk factors include diseases (Box 2) and drugs (Box 3) that are associated with secondary osteoporosis.

The North American Menopause Society's (NAMS) recommendations are similar to those of the AACE, but include testing of premenopausal women who have experienced low-trauma osteoporotic fractures or secondary causes of osteoporosis [18]. Testing of premenopausal women results in

---

Box 1. Guidelines for measurement of bone mineral density (Web sites)

American Association of Clinical Endocrinologists (www.aace.org/clin/guidelines)

International Society for Clinical Densitometry (www.iscd.org/Visitors/positions/OfficialPositionsText.cfm)

National Institutes of Health

National Osteoporosis Foundation (www.nof.org/professionals/clinical.htm)

North American Menopause Society (www.menopause.org/edumaterials/cliniciansguide)

United States Preventive Services Task Force (www.ahrq.gov/clinic/uspstf/uspsoste.htm)

Box 2. Diseases associated with secondary osteoporosis

Endocrine diseases
Hypogonadism
Hyperparathyroidism
Hyperthyroidism
Hypercortisolism
Hyperprolactinemia
Diabetes mellitus, type I

Gastrointestinal diseases
Inflammatory bowel disease
Malabsorption syndromes
Celiac disease
Chronic liver disease
Gastric bypass operations

Other chronic diseases
Chronic rheumatic disorders
Rheumatoid arthritis
Ankylosing spondylitis
Chronic obstructive pulmonary disease
Renal disorders
Renal tubular acidosis
Idiopathic hypercalciuria
Malignancy
Multiple myeloma
Metastatic disease
Infiltrative disorders
Systemic mastocytosis
Hereditary disorders of connective tissue
Osteogenesis imperfecta

Organ transplantation

Dietary disorders
Vitamin D deficiency and insufficiency
Calcium deficiency
Excessive alcohol intake
Anorexia nervosa
Total parenteral nutrition

---

a conundrum; the US Food and Drug Administration has not approved any medication for the treatment of osteoporosis in premenopausal women.

The ISCD recommends BMD testing using DXA in all postmenopausal women aged 65 years and older and in all men aged 70 years and older [4].

Box 3. Drugs associated with secondary osteoporosis

Glucocorticoids
Anticonvulsants
Excessive thyroid hormone replacement
Immunosuppressive agents
Heparin
GnRH antagonists
Depo-Provera
Drugs used to treat breast cancer
Tamoxifen (premenopausal women)
Aromatase inhibitors (postmenopausal women)

The ISCD also recommends BMD testing in younger postmenopausal women with risk factors, and in adult men and women who have diseases or conditions or are taking medications that are associated with low bone mass or bone loss. The ISCD is the only professional organization that has proposed recommendations for BMD testing in men.

Finally, the US Preventive Services Task Force has the most restricted guidelines; it recommends BMD testing in all postmenopausal women aged 65 years and older and in women aged 60 to 64 years with risk factors for fracture [19].

In addition to these clinical practice guidelines, several algorithms have been published that can be used to identify women who should undergo BMD testing [20–23]; these complement the clinical practice guidelines that are listed in Box 1 and were reviewed briefly above. These algorithms include the Osteoporosis Risk Assessment Index (ORAI), the Simple Calculated Osteoporosis Risk Equation (SCORE), and the Osteoporosis Self-Assessment Tool (OST); the OST also has been used in men [24]. The ORAI includes five questions, whereas the SCORE includes six questions; both of these require calculation of a score that leads to identification of individuals who should be referred for testing for osteoporosis. The OST uses a formula that is based solely on age and body weight, and it has been adopted by the State of Maryland's Osteoporosis Education and Prevention Task Force for identifying women and men who are at low, medium, or high risk for osteoporosis based on a BMD T-score of −2.5 or less [25].

Raisz [26], in reviewing these recommendations and algorithms, concluded that BMD measurements should be obtained routinely in all women older than 65 years and in men and younger women who have had a fragility fracture, have medical conditions, or are taking medications that are associated with secondary osteoporosis. In addition, he recommended measurement of BMD with DXA in women who have a T-score of −1.0 or less based on a peripheral densitometry measurement.

There is clear evidence that universal testing of women aged 60 years and older is associated with a reduced rate of fractures [27,28]. LaCroix and colleagues [27] randomized more than 9000 women, aged 60 to 80 years, who were not taking hormone therapy or other osteoporosis medications to one of three groups: universal testing (n = 1986), testing based on results of SCORE (n = 1940), and testing based on results of a 17-item questionnaire that was adapted from known risk factors for hip fracture (n = 5342). BMD measurements were performed in 415, 425, and 150 women in each group, respectively. During a mean follow-up of 33 months, the rate of osteoporotic fractures was 74.11, 99.44, and 91.77 per 1000 woman-years, respectively (P < .05 comparing the other two groups with the universal screening group). The rate of hip fractures also was lower in the universal screening group, but differences were not statistically significant (8.54, 9.04, and 13.31 per 1000 woman-years, respectively). These results were extended by an analysis of data from the Cardiovascular Health Study [28]. In this population-based observational cohort study, 1378 eligible participants who were enrolled in the Sacramento County (California) and Allegheny County (Pennsylvania) sites completed measurement of BMD at the hip, whereas 1685 participants who were enrolled in the Washington County (Maryland) and Forsyth County (North Carolina) sites received usual care. Mean age was 76 years, most were women, and more than 80% were white. The incidence of hip fractures over a mean of 4.9 years of follow-up was 4.8 and 8.2 per 1000 person-years in the screened and usual care group, respectively (multiple variable adjusted relative hazard, 0.64; 95% CI 0.41–0.99). There was no evidence of a statistical interaction between screening and sex, age group, or race; however, there were only four hip fractures in the 532 black participants (Blacks have a lower rate of hip fractures than do whites in both sexes). Hence, these two studies provide strong support for the recommendation of universal BMD testing that was summarized above.

Who should be treated to reduce fracture risk?

Lewiecki [15] identified 103 clinical practice guidelines for BMD treatment of osteoporosis. Of these, 3 were unique guidelines that fulfilled his inclusion/exclusion criteria and addressed treatment: those from the AACE, NAMS, and NOF [16–18]. All 3 are focused on treating postmenopausal women; the AACE and NAMS guidelines recommend treating women with a T-score measured by central DXA of −2.5 or less, whereas the NOF guidelines recommend treatment at a T-score of −2.0 or less. All modify the T-score cut-point in the presence of other risk factors for fracture, including a history of a low-trauma symptomatic fracture or a radiographic vertebral fracture. Hence, the NOF recommends treatment at a T-score of −1.5 or less in the presence of one or more risk factors, including a previous clinical fracture or radiographic vertebral fracture.

Solomon and colleagues [29] also performed a systematic review of the English-language literature using MEDLINE and HealthStar for the period between January 1992 and December 2003 to identify osteoporosis treatment guidelines. They identified 18 unique guidelines; 17 provided recommendations for postmenopausal women and 13 provided recommendations for men. Most osteoporosis treatment guidelines that included recommendations for postmenopausal women also suggested that treatment should be provided to women with BMD T-scores of less than −2.5 if other risk factors for fracture were present. The investigators concluded that existing clinical practice guidelines for treatment of osteoporosis presented a uniform series of recommendations.

Delmas and colleagues [30], in outlining the position of the International Osteoporosis Foundation, concluded that treatment of postmenopausal women who have established osteoporosis always is cost-effective and that additional scenarios exist when treatment is cost-effective. These additional scenarios depend upon the crossing of an "intervention threshold," where the future morbidity from osteoporotic fractures, largely derived from the costs of hip fracture, exceeds the costs of interventions that have been shown to reduce the risk for these fractures [31]. The "intervention threshold" probably will be defined based on the 10-year probability of fracture on a country-specific or health care system–specific basis, depending on cost-effectiveness thresholds. A working group of the World Health Organization, under the direction of Professor John Kanis of the University of Sheffield, England, has performed a series of meta-analyses to identify risk factors, independent of BMD, that contribute to the estimate of the 10-year fracture probability. The proposed risk factors include sex, age, history of fragility fracture [32], parental history of hip fracture [33], current smoking [34], use of systemic glucocorticoids [35], excess alcohol intake [36], and presence of rheumatoid arthritis; body mass index will be used in countries with limited or no access to BMD testing, because these are correlated highly [31]. Sex-specific algorithms are being developed by this group to allow calculation of person-specific 10-year fracture probability that can be applied on a country-specific basis to determine whether treatment is cost-effective in that specific health care system [37]. The NOF has established a working group to develop a questionnaire that can be administered at the time of BMD testing, so that the 10-year fracture risk can be estimated for each individual who undergoes a BMD test and recommendations can be made at the time of reporting results of the BMD test (E. Siris, MD, personal communication, 2006). The impact of this policy likely will become apparent over the remaining years of this decade.

Summary

Clinical practice guidelines exist for the diagnosis and treatment of osteoporosis in men and postmenopausal women. These guidelines present a uniform set of recommendations. Unfortunately, studies have shown a low rate of screening and treatment, particularly in high-risk groups, such as patients who have experienced a fracture. It is hoped that quality improvement projects, such as that being conducted by the American Medical Association in conjunction with numerous specialty societies, will lead to an improvement in physician practices in this area that will result in a reduction in morbidity and mortality from osteoporotic fractures.

References

[1] NIH Consensus Development Panel on Osteoporosis. Osteoporosis prevention, diagnosis and therapy. JAMA 2001;285:785–95.

[2] Cummings SR, Black DM, Nevitt MC, et al. Bone density at various sties for prediction of hip fractures. Lancet 1993;341:72–5.

[3] World Health Organization Study Group. Assessment of fracture risk and its application to screening for postmenopausal osteoporosis. World Health Organ Tech Rep Ser 1994;843: 1–129.

[4] Official positions of the International Society for Clinical Densitometry: Updated 2005. Available at: http://www.iscd.org. Accessed August 22, 2005.

[5] Kado KM, Browner WS, Palermo L, et al. Vertebral fractures and mortality in older women: a prospective study. Arch Intern Med 1999;159:1215–20.

[6] Ensrud KE, Thompson DE, Cauley JA, et al. Prevalent vertebral deformities predict mortality and hospitalization in older women with low bone mass: Fracture Intervention Trial Research Group. J Am Geriatr Soc 2000;48:241–9.

[7] Department of Health and Human Services. Bone health and osteoporosis: a report of the Surgeon General. Rockville, MD: Office of the Surgeon General; 2004.

[8] Cranney A, Guyatt G, Griffith L, et al. Meta-analyses of therapies for postmenopausal osteoporosis: IX. Summary of meta-analyses of therapies for postmenopausal osteoporosis. Endocr Rev 2002;23:570–8.

[9] Neer RM, Arnaud CD, Zanchetta JR, et al. Effect of parathyroid hormone (1–34) on fractures and bone mineral density in postmenopausal women with osteoporosis. N Engl J Med 2001;344:1434–41.

[10] Chesnut CH III, Skag A, Christiansen C, et al. Effects of oral ibandronate administered daily or intermittently on fracture risk in postmenopausal osteoporosis. J Bone Miner Res 2004; 19:1241–9.

[11] Orwoll E, Ettinger M, Weiss S, et al. Alendronate for the treatment of osteoporosis in men. N Engl J Med 2000;31(343):604–10.

[12] Kaufman JM, Orwoll E, Goemaere S, et al. Teriparatide effects on vertebral fractures and bone mineral density in men with osteoporosis: treatment and discontinuation of therapy. Osteoporos Int 2005;16:510–6.

[13] Morris CA, Cabrall D, Cheng H, et al. Patterns of bone mineral density testing: current guidelines, testing rates and interventions. J Gen Intern Med 2004;19(7):783–90.

[14] Elliot-Gibson V, Bogoch ER, Jamal SA, et al. Practice patterns in the diagnosis and treatment of osteoporosis after a fragility fracture: a systematic review. Osteoporos Int 2004; 15:767–78.

[15] Lewiecki EM. Review of guidelines for bone mineral density testing and treatment of osteoporosis. Curr Osteopor Rep 2005;3(3):75–83.

[16] National Osteoporosis Foundation. Osteoporosis: review of the evidence for prevention, diagnosis and treatment and cost-effectiveness analysis. Osteoporos Int 1998;8(Suppl 4): S7–80.

[17] Hodgson SF, Watts NB, Bilezikian JP, et al. American Association of Clinical Endocrinologists medical guidelines for clinical practice for the prevention and treatment of postmenopausal osteoporosis: 2001 edition, with selected updates for 2003. Endocrin Prac 2003;9: 544–64.

[18] North American Menopause Society. Management of postmenopausal osteoporosis: position statement of the North American Menopause Society. Menopause 2002;9(2): 84–101.

[19] US Preventive Services Task Force. Screening for osteoporosis in postmenopausal women: recommendations and rationale. Ann Intern Med 2002;137:526–8.

[20] Cadarette SM, Jaglal SB, Krieger N, et al. Development and validation of the Osteoporosis Risk Assessment Instrument to facilitate selection of women for bone densitometry. CMAJ 2000;162:1289–94.

[21] Lydick E, Cook K, Turpin J, et al. Development and validation of a simple questionnaire to facilitate identification of women likely to have low bone density. Am J Manag Care 1998;4: 37–48.

[22] Geusens P, Hochberg MC, van der Voort DJ, et al. Performance of risk indices for identifying low bone density in postmenopausal women. Mayo Clin Proc 2002;77:629–37.

[23] Cadarette SM, McIsaac WJ, Hawker GA, et al. The validity of decision rules for selecting women with primary osteoporosis for bone mineral density testing. Osteoporos Int 2004; 15:361–6.

[24] Adler R, Tran MT, Petkov VI. Performance of the osteoporosis self-assessment screening tool for osteoporosis in American men. Mayo Clin Proc 2003;78:723–7.

[25] Maryland Department of Health and Mental Hygiene Family Health Administration. Osteoporosis risk assessment in Maryland: Maryland Osteoporosis Prevention and Education Task Force Risk Assessment Workgroup Recommendations, 2004. Available at: http://www.strongerbones.org/tfworkgroups.html. Accessed August 22, 2005.

[26] Raisz LG. Screening for osteoporosis. N Engl J Med 2005;353:164–71.

[27] LaCroix AZ, Buist DSM, Brenneman SK, et al. Evaluation of three population-based strategies for fracture prevention: results of the Osteoporosis Population-Based Risk Assessment (OPRA) Trial. Med Care 2005;43:293–302.

[28] Kern LM, Powe NR, Levine MA, et al. Association between screening for osteoporosis and the incidence of hip fracture. Ann Intern Med 2005;142:173–81.

[29] Solomon DH, Morris C, Cheng H, et al. Medication use patterns for osteoporosis: an assessment of guidelines, treatment rates, and quality improvement interventions. Mayo Clin Proc 2005;80:194–202.

[30] Delmas PD, Rizzoli R, Cooper C, et al. Treatment of patients with postmenopausal osteoporosis is worthwhile: the position of the International Osteoporosis Foundation. Osteoporos Int 2005;16:1–5.

[31] Kanis JA, Borgstrom F, De Laet C, et al. Assessment of fracture risk. Osteoporos Int 2005; 16:581–9.

[32] Kanis JA, Johnell O, De Laet C, et al. A meta-analysis of previous fracture and subsequent fracture risk. Bone 2004;35:375–82.

[33] Kanis JA, Johansson H, Oden A, et al. A family history of fracture and fracture risk: a meta-analysis. Bone 2004;35:1029–37.

[34] Kanis JA, Johnell O, Oden A, et al. Smoking and fracture risk: a meta-analysis. Osteoporos Int 2005;16:155–62.

[35] Kanis JA, Johansson H, Johnell O, et al. Alcohol intake as a risk factor for fracture. Osteoporos Int 2005;16:737–42.

[36] Kanis JA, Johansson H, Oden A, et al. A meta-analysis of prior corticosteroid use and fracture risk. J Bone Miner Res 2004;19:893–9.

[37] De Laet C, Oden A, Johansson H, et al. The impact of the use of multiple risk indicators for fracture on case-finding strategies: a mathematical approach. Osteoporos Int 2005;16: 313–8.

ELSEVIER
SAUNDERS

RHEUMATIC
DISEASE CLINICS
OF NORTH AMERICA

Rheum Dis Clin N Am 32 (2006) 691–702

Emerging Issues With Bisphosphonates

Ian R. Reid, MD

Faculty of Medical and Health Sciences, University of Auckland,
Private Bag 92019, Auckland, New Zealand

The bisphosphonates are now the class of drugs most widely used in the treatment of osteoporosis, and they are also useful in many other conditions in which inhibition of osteoclastic bone resorption is desirable. The bisphosphonate nucleus consists of two phosphate groups linked through a central carbon atom. The negative charge on the phosphate groups gives this class of compounds a high affinity for the positively charged calcium ions on the surface of bone. The other side-chains attached to the central carbon atom distinguish the different members of the class from one another and determine the avidity of binding to the bone surface and the antiresorptive potency. From a functional point of view, the bisphosphonates may be divided into those that contain a nitrogen atom in their side-chain and those that do not (eg, etidronate, clodronate, tiludronate). The former are more potent and account for virtually all of the clinically used bisphosphonates at this time.

Pharmacology

The bisphosphonates have unique pharmacokinetics. Their propensity to bind to any positively charged species confers a low oral bioavailability (approximately 1%). If any intestinal absorption is to take place, they must be taken fasting, with water alone, separated by some hours from the ingestion of other charged compounds, such as calcium supplements and antacids. While passing through the stomach and esophagus, they can cause local irritation or ulceration, particularly if a patient who has gastro-esophageal reflux lies down after dosing. For these reasons, appropriate dosing procedures are critical to both the safety and efficacy of oral bisphosphonates. These problems have encouraged the intravenous

---

E-mail address: i.reid@auckland.ac.nz

administration of bisphosphonates, an approach that is facilitated by the long duration of action of these drugs.

Bisphosphonates in the circulation are either rapidly absorbed onto bone surfaces or excreted unmetabolized in the urine, in approximately equal proportions. It is widely believed that bisphosphonates taken up by bone are exclusively localized under resorbing osteoclasts [1]. However, there is compelling evidence that their deposition is much more widespread, including active and inactive bone surfaces [2]. The activity of osteoclasts is rapidly inhibited by their uptake of bisphosphonates, which results in inhibition of farnesyl diphosphate synthase, an enzyme in the mevalonate pathway that is important in the maintenance of the cytoskeleton and for cell survival. The presence of bisphosphonate on other bone surfaces provides a reservoir of the drug that, over the coming months and years, can poison future generations of osteoclasts that attempt to resorb these surfaces. It is likely that there is local reuptake of bisphosphonate released from bone, and limited local diffusion of bisphosphonate through bone has been hypothesized. As new bone is formed, previously deposited bisphosphonates become buried and unable to influence bone turnover, but they are potentially available many years later, when that newly formed packet of bone is eventually resorbed. Thus, with long-term use of bisphosphonates, a progressive labeling of the entire skeleton may well occur. This process will occur more rapidly in trabecular bone, because of its more rapid turnover.

Antifracture efficacy

The capacity of bisphosphonates to prevent fractures in osteoporotic women is now well established, particularly for alendronate and risedronate. The phase 3 alendronate trial [3] and both arms of the Fracture Intervention Trial [4,5] showed approximately 50% decreases in vertebral fractures, and the pooled estimate from all the alendronate trials is a relative risk for vertebral fracture of 0.52 (95% confidence interval [CI] 0.43–0.65) [6]. Clear evidence also indicates that alendronate decreases the risk for nonvertebral fractures in women who have osteoporosis, whether this is defined in terms of prevalent fracture or in terms of bone mineral density (BMD) [7]. This effect was first clearly demonstrated by Black and colleagues [4] and was subsequently independently confirmed by Pols and colleagues in a 1-year study [8]. The pooled relative risk for osteoporotic women estimated by Cranney is 0.49 (95% CI 0.36–0.67). The 10-year follow-up of the phase 3 study suggests that nonvertebral fractures remain reduced in those who continue to take alendronate, but the numbers of subjects are insufficient for certainty on this point [9].

Risedronate reduces vertebral fractures in osteoporotic women [10,11] (pooled relative risk 0.64, 95% CI 0.54–0.77 [12]), including those who do not have prevalent fractures [13]. Risedronate also reduces nonvertebral fractures: Harris and colleagues [10] found a decrease of 39% over 3 years, and McClung and colleagues [14] found a 30% reduction in hip fractures in a population of women older than 70 years. When available data on nonvertebral fractures are meta-analyzed, relative risk after treatment with risedronate is 0.73 (95% CI 0.61–0.87) [12]. Pooling of data from the risedronate studies indicates that reductions in both vertebral [15] and nonvertebral fractures [16] are apparent within 6 months of initiating treatment with this drug.

Oral ibandronate, used either continuously (2.5 mg/d) or intermittently (20 mg every other day for the first 24 days, followed by 9 weeks without active drug), produces changes in BMD comparable to those found with oral alendronate or risedronate [17]. A weekly dose of 20 mg appears to be similarly effective [18,19]. Both the daily and cyclic regimens have now been shown to reduce vertebral fractures by about one half, but nonvertebral fractures were only reduced in a post-hoc analysis that was restricted to those who had femoral neck T-scores of less than −3 [20]. Intravenous ibandronate 3 mg, every 3 months produces similar changes in BMD [21,22], but its antifracture efficacy is unknown.

This review of fracture data indicates that antifracture efficacy has only been demonstrated for a limited number of regimens, many of which are no longer in routine clinical use. Thus, alendronate and risedronate are now usually given weekly, and ibandronate is coming into use as a monthly tablet or less frequent intravenous injection. No antifracture data exist for any of these regimens, which have been registered on the basis that they produce comparable effects on BMD and bone turnover to the daily oral use of the respective drugs. Considering the difficulty and expense involved in demonstrating antifracture efficacy, this use of surrogate endpoints is probably appropriate. However, it does raise the broader question of whether any bisphosphonate that meets comparable density and turnover criteria should also be licensed for clinical use. This is certainly not the current view of the regulatory agencies, but it appears to be a reasonable way to proceed on the basis of our understanding of the biology involved.

Fracture prevention in osteopenic women

Bisphosphonates have positive effects on BMD in women who do not have osteoporosis. For example, in a study of recently menopausal women, alendronate treatment for 7 years increased spine and trochanter BMD by 3% to 4%, while femoral neck BMD was maintained [23]. A 2-year study with risedronate produced similar results [24]. An important unresolved issue is that of whether bisphosphonates prevent fractures in individuals who do not already have osteoporosis. Studies with both alendronate [5] and risedronate [14] have suggested that they do not, although neither of these studies was powered specifically to address this issue. The findings of the Women's Health Initiative suggest that estrogen/progestin prevents

fractures in unselected older women, and a recent study comparing clodronate 800 mg/d with placebo in 5592 women aged 75 years or older also
found 20% fewer clinical fractures over 3 years [25]. Antifracture efficacy
was independent of age, body mass index, baseline BMD, and prior fracture
history. This finding represents a potentially significant expansion of the indications for use of bisphosphonates, particularly as the advent of generics
renders them more affordable.

Differences among bisphosphonates

Major differences clearly exist among bisphosphonates in their antiresorptive potency, zoledronate being more than 100,000 times more potent
in some assays than the first agent in clinical use, etidronate. The clinical
usefulness of etidronate was limited by its interference with bone mineralization when given continuously in doses that produced clinically useful
inhibition of bone resorption. The newer agents have much lower potency
in the inhibition of mineralization and a much higher antiresorptive
potency, so they are effectively free of mineralization-inhibiting properties
at clinically used doses.

Until recently, it was believed that the nitrogen-containing bisphosphonates were therapeutically equivalent to one another when used in doses
that produce the same antiresorptive effects. This concept is now being
challenged, partially on the basis of scientific evidence and partially as
a commercial strategy by pharmaceutical companies that wish to create
a unique profile for their particular product and rebut any perception that
their drug is simply a "metoodronate." Some objective data support the
distinctions being made between the various compounds. For instance, risedronate is approximately five times more potent than alendronate as an
inhibitor of farnesyl diphosphate synthase, but it is used in clinical practice
in a dose only one half that of alendronate. Even at this dose, it produces
smaller increments in bone density and less marked suppression of bone resorption than does alendronate [26]. Similarly, intravenous doses of ibandronate wear off in less than 3 months [27,28], whereas a single dose of
zoledronate can last for more than 1 year [29]. This apparent contrast
may have two explanations. First, there has been a recent focus on the
capacity and avidity of the binding of bisphosphonates to bone. In vitro
studies suggest that zoledronate and alendronate show much tighter binding
to hydroxyapatite than other bisphosphonates [30]. This effect would
theoretically lead to increased uptake of the drug by bone and a more
prolonged duration of action.

A second mechanism may underlie some of the apparent differences in
duration of action in clinical studies, namely, the same degree of inhibition
of bone resorption was not achieved with the doses being compared. This
factor is certainly relevant to the duration of action of ibandronate, which
is significantly longer when larger doses that achieve more marked

suppression of turnover are used. This aspect may also underlie the apparent differences between the rates of offset of risedronate and alendronate, because alendronate in conventional doses suppresses turnover to a greater extent.

The available human data are difficult to interpret, because none of them are head-to-head comparisons in which comparable inhibition of bone turnover has been achieved. Two animal studies potentially address this point. Gasser and colleagues [31] have shown that the offset of changes in bone mineral density following single injections of alendronate, risedronate, ibandronate, and zoledronate is the same if the same initial therapeutic response is achieved. In contrast, Fuchs and colleagues [32] have shown a more rapid offset of the effect of risedronate on trabecular bone turnover than was seen after alendronate, when the two agents were given in doses that achieved the same inhibition of turnover. In the Fuchs study, the medication was administered over a period of 8 weeks, suggesting that mode and duration of administration may influence the rate of offset.

How long should bisphosphonates be continued in osteoporosis?

Since the introduction of bisphosphonates, there has been concern that these potent antiresorptives would decrease bone turnover to a level where microdamage would not be repaired, resulting in decreased biomechanical strength. Although such effects have been demonstrated in animal models treated with high doses of bisphosphonates [33], this phenomenon has not been found in human studies, where, in contrast, fracture rates are found to decrease. Isolated reports of stress fractures [34] or delayed healing of fractures [35] in patients treated with bisphosphonates have appeared. In the absence of persuasive control data, the consensus is that this is not a major issue within the periods covered by controlled trials and their extensions. However, this does not mean that microdamage accumulation will not become a problem with very long-term therapy, so many authorities believe that it is sensible to consider limiting the duration of use of these drugs in some way.

The idea of a drug holiday or dose reduction with long-term use is made more acceptable by the evidence that the effects of some agents persist after their discontinuation. When alendronate is discontinued, bone turnover rises to some extent, but even several years after the end of long-term use, bone resorption rates have not returned to baseline [9,36,37]. Preliminary data have been presented suggesting that the offset of risedronate's effect is more rapid. But the degree of suppression was less than that in the alendronate studies, so these data are not directly comparable [24,38]. Greenspan and colleagues [39] found that there was a significant loss of BMD after the termination of 2 years of treatment with estrogen/progestin, whereas no such loss was seen following termination of a similar period of treatment with alendronate. McClung [37] found that there was some loss of BMD following 2 or 4 years of therapy with alendronate, but this loss was again much smaller than that following a similar period of treatment with estrogen/progestin. Bagger and colleagues [36] assessed women 7 years after alendronate withdrawal and found that those who received alendronate (2.5 to 10 mg per day) for 2 years had a 3.8% higher BMD than those who received placebo. The residual effect was proportionally larger in women who had received treatment for longer periods (4 years, 5.9%, $P = .02$; 6 years, 8.6%, $P = .002$).

The 10-year follow-up of the phase 3 alendronate study suggests that non-vertebral fractures remain reduced in those who continue to take alendronate, but the numbers of subjects were insufficient for certainty on this point [9]. The Fracture Intervention Trial has also been extended: 1099 women who were assigned to active therapy in the Fracture Intervention Trial and had an average duration of alendronate use of 5 years were rerandomized to alendronate (30% to 10 mg/d, 30% to 5 mg/d) or to placebo (40% of the cohort) for an additional 5 years. Preliminary data for the 5-year endpoint of this extension [40] show relative risks for clinical spine fracture of 0.45 and for nonspine fracture of 1.0, when those continuing on either dose of alendronate are compared with those receiving placebo. The two doses appeared to perform comparably. This finding indicates that continuation of alendronate for 10 years produces marginally more beneficial fracture outcomes than does its discontinuation after only 5 years, but there is no evidence of a waning of effect or development of increased skeletal fragility. Discontinuation of risedronate after 3 years is followed by persistence of the low fracture rates in the following year [41], and continuation of risedronate to 7 years is also associated with maintenance of low fracture rates [42].

On the basis of these findings, several courses are open. One is to conclude that treatment for as long as 10 years is safe and effective and to continue treatment for most patients for this period. This course is supported by both the extended studies of alendronate. In women who are taking alendronate, a second option is to reduce the dose from 10 mg/d to 5 mg/d (or its equivalent) after 5 years of use. This course is consistent with the Fracture Intervention Trial extension, which does not show a fracture advantage of alendronate 10 mg/d over 5 mg/d during the second quinquennium of treatment, although a detailed breakdown of the data by dose is not yet available. Whether such a dose reduction is appropriate for risedronate cannot be determined. A third course is suggested by the recent analysis of the relationship between fracture incidence and bone resorption in the risedronate studies [43]. This analysis suggests that the intermittent use of bisphosphonates to maintain resorption markers 1.5 standard deviations below the premenopausal mean may produce optimal fracture prevention. However, available data do not address this issue in the context of use for 5 to 10 years or in direct comparison with other treatment strategies.

In recent years, it has been generally accepted that the surrogate endpoints of BMD and bone turnover do not guarantee antifracture efficacy.

Therefore, it is not possible to determine which of the approaches described here is optimal in terms of the one endpoint that really matters, namely fracture. The least speculative course is to continue bisphosphonate until year 10 and then consider dose reduction along with monitoring of BMD and turnover. Unfortunately, there is no prospect of authoritative data beyond 10 years becoming available in the foreseeable future.

Combining other agents with bisphosphonates

In an effort to increase efficacy, combinations of bisphosphonates with a number of other agents have been assessed. For instance, Lindsay and colleagues [44] have shown that the addition of alendronate to pre-existing hormone therapy leads to further suppression of bone resorption markers and increases in BMD. Harris and colleagues [45] conducted a head-to-head trial of risedronate plus estrogen versus estrogen alone. Again, a greater suppression of bone resorption was found in the combined therapy group, with a marginal benefit in terms of additional BMD gain of approximately 1%. Similar data indicate additivity of effects of bisphosphonates with ralox-ifene [46]. It is unknown whether the marginally greater antiresorptive effects that come from combination therapy result in any greater effect on fracture.

Greater interest has developed in the possible additivity of bisphospho-nates with an anabolic agent such as parathyroid hormone (PTH). The use of PTH in women who have already been taking estrogen for some time re-sults in substantial further gains in BMD [47], as it does after raloxifene [48]. However, the anabolic response appears to be substantially blunted in patients previously treated with alendronate [48]. When alendronate and PTH are initiated at the same time, combination therapy results in changes in markers and BMD that are intermediate between those seen in subjects receiving monotherapy with either agent alone [49,50]. Gasser and colleagues [51] have recently found that a single intravenous dose of bisphosphonate before the initiation of PTH permits a fully additive BMD response to the combined therapy, by contrast with the situation of oral dosing.

A third way of combining a bisphosphonate with PTH is to give the PTH first, followed by the bisphosphonate. Black and colleagues [52] have recently described such a regimen. Women who had been treated with PTH for a year were then randomized to continue on placebo or alendro-nate, the PTH being discontinued in both groups. In the subsequent year, there were substantially more positive changes in BMD in those who started on alendronate. Thus, PTH followed by bisphosphonate appears to be the optimal combination, but there is clearly more work to be done in this area.

Bisphosphonates in Paget's disease

Although bisphosphonates are most widely used in osteoporosis, it is important to remember that they are crucial to the management of other bone conditions as well. Paget's disease is a focal or multifocal abnormality of greatly increased bone turnover. It is therefore ideally suited to therapy with bisphosphonates, and these drugs have revolutionized its management. Bisphosphonates are taken up more avidly in sites of high bone turnover; hence they are effectively targeted to the pagetic lesions.

For reasons that are largely historical, bisphosphonates tend to be given as courses in Paget's disease. A course may comprise one or more injections of an agent such as pamidronate, or 2 to 6 months of daily administration of an oral medication (as for risedronate and alendronate, respectively). The latest generation of potent intravenous bisphosphonates offers the possibility of more complete and longer-lasting control of pagetic activity. The author and colleagues [53] have recently explored this using both ibandronate and zoledronate. One or two 6-mg injections of ibandronate were similarly effective, reducing alkaline phosphatase levels by 70% and resulting in normalization or near-normalization of bone scintigrams in 60% of patients. The phase 3 zoledronate program compared a single infusion of zoledronate, 5 mg, with 2 months of daily oral risedronate (30 mg/d) [54]. Both agents produced substantial therapeutic benefits, with normalization of alkaline phosphatase in 89% and 58% of patients for zoledronate and risedronate, respectively. Ongoing follow-up of these study patients has shown a dramatic divergence between the two therapies. Thus, at a median follow-up of 26 months from the beginning of the study, only three of the 152 patients who showed a significant response to zoledronate have lost this response, whereas more than 50% of those responding to risedronate no longer show a clinical response.

The present data pose the question of how the choice should be made between oral and intravenous bisphosphonates in treating Paget's disease. The key issue is that, whichever potent bisphosphonate is used, it should be given with a clear therapeutic endpoint in mind and in a dose and duration adequate to achieve that endpoint. Whether an oral or intravenous agent is used is largely a question of the personal preference of the patient. Those who have a history of upper gastrointestinal problems or who find difficulties with the restrictions imposed by daily dosing with oral bisphosphonates will favor an intravenous agent. By contrast, those who have experienced severe acute phase reactions with parenteral bisphosphonates or who are unwilling to accept the discomfort of intravenous injections will opt for longer-term oral dosing. As long as the supervising physician has a clear therapeutic endpoint in mind at the outset, an adequate outcome should be achieved with either class of agent. Current evidence suggests that zoledronate may achieve longer-lasting remissions than the other available agents.

No universal consensus exists regarding the indications for treatment of Paget's disease. As in the studies reviewed earlier, surrogate endpoints (usually biochemical) have been used in most assessments of therapies for this condition, and there is no clinical trial evidence that antipagetic therapy can prevent the progression of deformity, the development of pagetic symptoms, or fracture. However, it is clear that treating Paget's disease leads to a restoration of normal bone histology [55], that it can lead to the healing of lytic lesions on radiographs [55], and that, in the absence of such intervention, both bone lysis and deformity progress. In the absence of clinical trial data that address these important questions (and given the unlikelihood of such data's becoming available), it appears unreasonable to withhold safe therapies that are able to halt histologic and radiologic disease progression. Therefore, many experienced physicians endorse the provision of antipagetic therapy to individuals who have lytic lesions in long bones, lesions at sites that are likely to lead to neurologic complications, arthritis, or deformity, or involvement of the skull that could compromise hearing [56,57].

Osteonecrosis of the jaw

Osteonecrosis of the jaw is a new clinical entity for most doctors [58], which may be related to sustained and substantial inhibition of bone turnover. It presents as an area of exposed, necrotic bone in either the mandible or maxilla, which persists for a number of months. This problem is being recognized in oncology patients, many of whom have been treated with high-dose monthly bisphosphonates. It is most commonly seen in those who have metastatic breast cancer or multiple myeloma. The possible association with the use of bisphosphonates has raised the issue of whether this is a problem in those who use bisphosphonates for benign indications, such as osteoporosis and Paget's disease. Some case reports of this phenomenon now exist, although they constitute only a few percent of the total number of cases recorded. Approximately 100 cases have been reported worldwide with alendronate, in the context of 20 million patient-years of use of this drug.

The lesions develop following major dental procedures, such as extractions or dental implants, although they are sometimes associated with local trauma from dentures. Some dentists recommend that such procedures be entirely avoided in those who have a history of bisphosphonate use. To many working in the field, this appears to be an overreaction to what is, outside the context of oncology practice, a very rare event. Although the pathogenesis and causation of this condition are being further explored, it does appear cautious to carry out any planned major dental procedures *before* individuals start taking bisphosphonates. However, it must be borne in mind that substantial delays in the initiation of bisphosphonate therapy in those who are at a substantial risk for fracture will lead to the occurrence of preventable fractures.

References

[1] Sato M, Grasser W, Endo N, et al. Bisphosphonate action. Alendronate localization in rat bone and effects on osteoclast ultrastructure. J Clin Invest 1991;88(6):2095–105.

[2] Masarachia P, Weinreb M, Balena R, et al. Comparison of the distribution of 3H-alendronate and 3H-etidronate in rat and mouse bones. Bone 1996;19(3):281–90.

[3] Liberman UA, Weiss SR, Broll J, et al. Effect of oral alendronate on bone mineral density and the incidence of fractures in postmenopausal osteoporosis. N Engl J Med 1995; 333(22):1437–43.

[4] Black DM, Cummings SR, Karpf DB, et al. Randomised trial of effect of alendronate on risk of fracture in women with existing vertebral fractures. Lancet 1996;348(9041):1535–41.

[5] Cummings SR, Black DM, Thompson DE, et al. Effect of alendronate on risk of fracture in women with low bone density but without vertebral fractures—results from the Fracture Intervention Trial. JAMA 1998;280(24):2077–82.

[6] Cranney A, Wells G, Willan A, et al. Meta-analysis of alendronate for the treatment of postmenopausal women. Endocr Rev 2002;23(4):508–16.

[7] Black DM, Thompson DE, Bauer DC, et al. Fracture risk reduction with alendronate in women with osteoporosis: the Fracture Intervention Trial. J Clin Endocrinol Metab 2000; 85(11):4118–24.

[8] Pols HAP, Felsenberg D, Hanley DA, et al. Multinational, placebo-controlled, randomized trial of the effects of alendronate on bone density and fracture risk in postmenopausal women with low bone mass: results of the FOSIT study. Osteoporos Int 1999;9(5):461–8.

[9] Bone HG, Hosking D, Devogelaer J, et al. Ten years' experience with alendronate for osteoporosis in postmenopausal women. N Engl J Med 2004;350(12):1189–99.

[10] Harris ST, Watts NB, Genant HK, et al. Effects of risedronate treatment on vertebral and nonvertebral fractures in women with postmenopausal osteoporosis—a randomized controlled trial. JAMA 1999;282(14):1344–52.

[11] Reginster JY, Minne HW, Sorensen OH, et al. Randomized trial of the effects of risedronate on vertebral fractures in women with established postmenopausal osteoporosis. Osteoporos Int 2000;11(1):83–91.

[12] Cranney A, Tugwell P, Adachi J, et al. Meta-analysis of risedronate for the treatment of postmenopausal osteoporosis. Endocr Rev 2002;23(4):517–23.

[13] Heaney RP, Zizic TM, Fogelman I, et al. Risedronate reduces the risk of first vertebral fracture in osteoporotic women. Osteoporos Int 2002;13(6):501–5.

[14] McClung MR, Geusens P, Miller PD, et al. Effect of risedronate on the risk of hip fracture in elderly women. N Engl J Med 2001;344(5):333–40.

[15] Roux C, Seeman E, Eastell R, et al. Efficacy of risedronate on clinical vertebral fractures within six months. Curr Med Res Opin 2004;20(4):433–9.

[16] Harrington JT, Ste-Marie LG, Brandi ML, et al. Risedronate rapidly reduces the risk for nonvertebral fractures in women with postmenopausal osteoporosis. Calcif Tissue Int 2004;74(2):129–35.

[17] Riis BJ, Ise J, Von Stein T, et al. Ibandronate: a comparison of oral daily dosing versus intermittent dosing in postmenopausal osteoporosis. J Bone Miner Res 2001;16(10):1871–8.

[18] Cooper C, Emkey RD, McDonald RH, et al. Efficacy and safety of oral weekly ibandronate in the treatment of postmenopausal osteoporosis. J Clin Endocrinol Metab 2003;88(10): 4609–15.

[19] Tanko LB, Felsenberg D, Czerwinski E, et al. Oral weekly ibandronate prevents bone loss in postmenopausal women. J Intern Med 2003;254(2):159–67.

[20] Chesnut CH, Skag A, Christiansen C. Effects of oral ibandronate administered daily or intermittently on fracture risk in postmenopausal osteoporosis. J Bone Miner Res 2004;19: 1241–9.

[21] Schimmer RC, Bauss F. Effect of daily and intermittent use of ibandronate on bone mass and bone turnover in postmenopausal osteoporosis: a review of three phase II studies. Clin Ther 2003;25(1):19–34.

[22] Adami S, Felsenberg D, Christiansen C, et al. Efficacy and safety of ibandronate given by intravenous injection once every 3 months. Bone 2004;34(5):881–9.

[23] Sambrook PN, Rodriguez JP, Wasnich RD, et al. Alendronate in the prevention of osteoporosis: 7-year follow-up. Osteoporos Int 2004;15(6):483–8.

[24] Mortensen L, Charles P, Bekker PJ, et al. Risedronate increases bone mass in an early postmenopausal population—two years of treatment plus one year of follow-up. J Clin Endocrinol Metab 1998;83(2):396–402.

[25] McCloskey E, Jalava T, Oden A, et al. The efficacy of clodronate (Bonefos®) to reduce the incidence of osteoporotic fractures in elderly women is independent of the underlying BMD. J Bone Miner Res 2003;18(Suppl 2):S92.

[26] Rosen CJ, Hochberg MC, Bonnick SL, et al. Treatment with once-weekly alendronate 70 mg compared with once-weekly risedronate 35 mg in women with postmenopausal osteoporosis: a randomized double-blind study. J Bone Miner Res 2005;20(1):141–51.

[27] Recker R, Stakkestad JA, Chesnut CH, et al. Insufficiently dosed intravenous ibandronate injections are associated with suboptimal antifracture efficacy in postmenopausal osteoporosis. Bone 2004;34(5):890–9.

[28] Christiansen C, Tanko LB, Warming L, et al. Dose dependent effects on bone resorption and formation of intermittently administered intravenous ibandronate. Osteoporos Int 2003; 14(7):609–13.

[29] Reid IR, Brown JP, Burckhardt P, et al. Intravenous zoledronic acid in postmenopausal women with low bone mineral density. N Engl J Med 2002;346(9):653–61.

[30] Nancollas GH, Tang R, Phipps RJ, et al. Novel insights into actions of bisphosphonates on bone: differences in interactions with hydroxyapatite. Bone 2006;38(5):617–27.

[31] Gasser J, Ingold P, Green J. A single IV injection of equipotent doses of alendronate, risedronate, ibandronate and zoledronic acid exerts a bone protective effect of similar magnitude and duration in ovariectomized rats. J Bone Miner Res 2004;19(Suppl 1):S307.

[32] Fuchs RK, Phipps RJ, Burr D. Trabecular bone turnover is reestablished sooner in ovariectomized rats after withdrawal of treatment with risedronate vs alendronate. Bone 2006; 38(3 Suppl 1):S50.

[33] Mashiba T, Hirano T, Turner CH, et al. Suppressed bone turnover by bisphosphonates increases microdamage accumulation and reduces some biomechanical properties in dog rib. J Bone Miner Res 2000;15(4):613–20.

[34] Guanabens N, Peris P, Monegal A, et al. Lower extremity stress fractures during intermittent cyclical etidronate treatment for osteoporosis. Calcif Tissue Int 1994;54(5):431–4.

[35] Odvina CV, Zerwekh JE, Rao DS, et al. Severely suppressed bone turnover: a potential complication of alendronate therapy. J Clin Endocrinol Metab 2005;90(3):1294–301.

[36] Bagger YZ, Tanko LB, Alexandersen P, et al. Alendronate has a residual effect on bone mass in postmenopausal Danish women up to 7 years after treatment withdrawal. Bone 2003; 33(3):301–7.

[37] McClung M. Resolution of effect following alendronate: six-year results from the Early Postmenopausal Interventional Cohort (EPIC) Study. J Bone Miner Res 2002;17(Suppl 1):S134.

[38] Watts NB, Olszynski W, McKeever C. Effect of risedronate treatment discontinuation on bone turnover and BMD. Calcif Tissue Int 2004;74(Suppl 1):S79.

[39] Greenspan SL, Emkey RD, Bone HG, et al. Significant differential effects of alendronate, estrogen, or combination therapy on the rate of bone loss after discontinuation of treatment of postmenopausal osteoporosis—a randomized, double-blind, placebo-controlled trial. Ann Intern Med 2002;137(11):875–83.

[40] Black D, Schwartz A, Ensrud K, et al. A 5 year randomized trial of the long-term efficacy and safety of alendronate: the FIT Long-term EXtension (FLEX). J Bone Miner Res 2004; 19(Suppl 1):S45.

[41] Watts NB, Barton IP, Olszynski WP, et al. Sustained reduction of vertebral fracture risk in the year after discontinuation of risedronate treatment. Osteoporos Int 2005;16(Suppl 3):S7.

[42] Goemaere S, Sorensen OH, Johnson TD, et al. Sustained anti-fracture efficacy of risedronate treatment over 7 years in postmenopausal women. J Bone Miner Res 2003;18(Suppl 2):S90.

[43] Eastell R, Barton I, Hannon RA, et al. Relationship of early changes in bone resorption to the reduction in fracture risk with risedronate. J Bone Miner Res 2003;18(6):1051–6.

[44] Lindsay R, Cosman F, Lobo RA, et al. Addition of alendronate to ongoing hormone replacement therapy in the treatment of osteoporosis: a randomized, controlled clinical trial. J Clin Endocrinol Metab 1999;84(9):3076–81.

[45] Harris ST, Eriksen EF, Davidson M, et al. Effect of combined risedronate and hormone replacement therapies on bone mineral density in postmenopausal women. J Clin Endocrinol Metab 2001;86(5):1890–7.

[46] Johnell O, Scheele WH, Lu YL, et al. Additive effects of raloxifene and alendronate on bone density and biochemical markers of bone remodeling in postmenopausal women with osteoporosis. J Clin Endocrinol Metab 2002;87(3):985–92.

[47] Lindsay R, Nieves J, Formica C, et al. Randomised controlled study of effect of parathyroid hormone on vertebral-bone mass and fracture incidence among postmenopausal women on oestrogen with osteoporosis. Lancet 1997;350(9077):550–5.

[48] Ettinger B, San Martin J, Crans G, et al. Differential effects of teriparatide on BMD after treatment with raloxifene or alendronate. J Bone Miner Res 2004;19(5):745–51.

[49] Black DM, Greenspan SL, Ensrud KE, et al. The effects of parathyroid hormone and alendronate alone or in combination in postmenopausal osteoporosis. N Engl J Med 2003;349(13):1207–15.

[50] Finkelstein JS, Hayes A, Hunzelman JL, et al. The effects of parathyroid hormone, alendronate, or both in men with osteoporosis. N Engl J Med 2003;349(13):1216–26.

[51] Gasser J, Ingold P, Rebmann A, et al. Inhibition of FPP-synthase in osteoblasts may explain the blunting of the bone anabolic response to PTH observed after chronic exposure of rats to bisphosphonates. Bone 2006;38(3 Suppl 1):S50.

[52] Black DM, Bilezikian JP, Ensrud KE, et al. One year of alendronate after one year of parathyroid hormone (1-84) for osteoporosis. N Engl J Med 2005;353(6):555–65.

[53] Reid IR, Davidson JS, Wattie D, et al. Comparative responses of bone turnover markers to bisphosphonate therapy in Paget's disease of bone. Bone 2004;35(1):224–30.

[54] Reid IR, Miller P, Lyles K, et al. Comparison of a single infusion of zoledronic acid with risedronate for Paget's disease. N Engl J Med 2005;353(9):898–908.

[55] Reid IR, Nicholson GC, Weinstein RS, et al. Biochemical and radiologic improvement in Paget's disease of bone treated with alendronate—a randomized, placebo-controlled trial. Am J Med 1996;101(4):341–8.

[56] Lyles KW, Siris ES, Singer FR, et al. A clinical approach to diagnosis and management of Paget's disease of bone. J Bone Miner Res 2001;16(8):1379–87.

[57] Delmas PD, Meunier PJ. The management of Paget's disease of bone. N Engl J Med 1997;336(8):558–66.

[58] Migliorati CA, Casiglia J, Epstein J, et al. Managing the care of patients with bisphosphonate-associated osteonecrosis—an American Academy of Oral Medicine position paper. J Am Dent Assoc 2005;136(12):1658–68.

**ELSEVIER
SAUNDERS**

RHEUMATIC
DISEASE CLINICS
OF NORTH AMERICA

Rheum Dis Clin N Am 32 (2006) 703–719

Parathyroid Hormone Update

Kendal L. Hamann, MD[a,b,]*, Nancy E. Lane, MD[c]

[a]*Division of Endocrinology, Clinical Nutrition, and Vascular Medicine, University of
California Davis Medical Center, 4150 V Street, Suite G400, Sacramento, CA 95817, USA*
[b]*Sacramento Mather Veterans' Affairs Medical Center, 10535 Hospital Way,
Mather Air Force Base, Mather, CA 95655, USA*
[c]*Department of Internal Medicine, University of California Davis Medical Center,
4800 2nd Avenue, Suite 2600 Sacramento, CA 95817, USA*

Osteoporosis afflicts an estimated 10 million United States citizens, and approximately one in two women and one in four men over the age of 50 will suffer from an osteoporosis-related fracture in their remaining lifetimes [1]. US Food and Drug Administration (FDA)-approved therapies for the treatment and prevention of osteoporosis include calcium and vitamin D supplements and antiresorptive therapies, such as bisphosphonates, estrogen, selective estrogen receptor modulators, and calcitonin. Recombinant human parathyroid hormone (rhPTH) and recombinant bioactive fragments of human parathyroid hormone are emerging as a unique new class of treatment options for osteoporosis. They are the only anabolic (as opposed to antiresorptive) agents available for clinical use. In 2002 the FDA approved teriparatide, a recombinant form of the N-terminal of endogenous human PTH known as rhPTH (1-34), for patients who have osteoporosis and are at high risk for fracture. A new drug application for the full-length recombinant peptide rhPTH (1-84) is under review with the FDA. This article briefly reviews the physiology and rationale for the use of PTH for the treatment of osteoporosis, and provides a more detailed update on the application of recent clinical trials of PTH to clinical practice. Table 1 summarizes the outcomes of recent clinical trials of PTH in human subjects.

Nancy Lane's work on this project is supported by the following grants from the National Institutes of Health: K24-ARO48841; RO1-AR43052.

* Corresponding author. Division of Endocrinology, UC Davis Medical Center, 4150 V Street, Suite G400, Sacramento, California 95817.

E-mail address: kendal.hamann@ucdmc.ucdavis.edu (K.L. Hamann).

Table 1
Summary of clinical trials for rPTH

Investigators	Population	Intervention	Effect on BMD	Effect on fracture risk
Neer et al DB, PC	1637 postmenopausal women with osteoporosis	20 or 40 µg rhPTH (1-34) vs. placebo; 21 mo.	Increase at LS, TH, and FN	65%–69% risk reduction vertebral fractures; 35%–40% risk reduction nonvertebral fractures.
Hodsman et al DB, PC	106 postmenopausal women with osteoporosis	50, 75, or 100 µg rhPTH (1-84) vs. placebo; 12 mo.	Increased at LS	N/A
Ettinger et al DB, PC	2532 postmenopausal women with osteoporosis	100 µg rhPTH (1-84) vs. placebo; 18 mo.	Increased at LS, TH, and FN	63%–66% risk reduction in vertebral fractures
Orwoll et al DB, PC	437 men with T scores < −2.0	20 or 40 µg rhPTH (1-34) vs. placebo; 11 mo.	Increased at LS and FN	N/A
Kurland et al DB, PC	23 men with osteoporosis	25 µg hPTH (1-34) vs. placebo; 18 mo.	Increased at LS and FN	N/A
Lane et al	51 postmenopausal women with osteoporosis on HRT and chronic steroids	25 µg hPTH (1-34) vs. placebo; 12 mo. treatment, 24 mo. follow-up.	Increased at LS: delayed increased at FN and TH 1 y after treatment.	N/A
Black et al (year 1) DB, PC	238 postmenopausal women with osteoporosis or at high risk	100 µg rhPTH (1-84) vs. combination with alendronate vs. alendronate alone; 12 mo.	Equally increased at LS in the rhPTH and combination groups	N/A
Finkelstein et al DB, PC	83 men with T scores < −2.0	40 µg hPTH (1-34) vs. combination with alendronate vs. alendronate alone; 30 mo.	Increased at LS and FN in the PTH-alone group	N/A

Rittmaster et al (uncontrolled)	66 postmenopausal women with osteoporosis	50, 75, or 100 μg rhPTH (1-84) vs. placebo for 1 y followed by 1 y alendronate	Increased at LS, FN, and TH on rhPTH followed by alendronate	N/A
Black et al (year 2) DB, PC	119 postmenopausal women after 1 y of rhPTH (1-84).	Second year of alendronate vs. placebo	Increased at LS and TH with subsequent alendronate; loss of BMD at the LS with subsequent placebo.	N/A
Cosman et al	126 women with osteoporosis previously on bisphosphonate therapy	25 μg daily vs. intermittent hPTH (1-34) combined with alendronate vs. alendronate alone; 12 mo.	Increased at LS in continuous and cyclic hPTH and alendronate combination groups	N/A
Lindsay et al	34 postmenopausal women with osteoporosis on HRT for at least 2 y	25 μg hPTH (1-34) plus HRT vs. HRT alone; 3 y.	Increased at LS and TH in the combination group	Less loss of vertebral height in the combination group
Cosman et al	52 postmenopausal women with osteoporosis on HRT for at least 1 y	25 μg hPTH (1-34) plus HRT vs. HRT alone; 3 y.	Increased at LS, TH in the combination group	Less loss of vertebral height in the combination group
Deal et al DB, PC	137 postmenopausal women with osteoporosis	20 μg rhPTH (1-34) alone vs. rhPTH plus raloxifene; 6 mo.	Increased at TH in the combination group	N/A

Abbreviations: BMD, bone mineral density; DB, double blinded; FN, femoral neck; hPTH, synthetic human parathyroid hormone; HRT, hormone replacement therapy with estrogen; LS, lumbar spine; PC, placebo controlled; rhPTH, recombinant human parathyroid hormone; TH, total hip.

Parathyroid hormone physiology

PTH is the principle regulator of calcium homeostasis. Its release from the parathyroid glands is triggered by hypocalcemia, and hypercalcemia suppresses its secretion. PTH stimulates osteoblast activity, increases gastrointestinal absorption of calcium, increases renal tubular reabsorption of calcium, and stimulates conversion of 25-hydroxyvitamin D to 1,25-dihydroxyvitamin D by 1-alpha hydroxylase in the kidney. The latter process further increases gastrointestinal absorption of calcium. Daily injection of PTH in animal models stimulates bone formation; however, continuously high levels of PTH as seen in clinical hyperparathyroidism usually result in diminished bone mineral density (BMD) over time. A clear threshold minimum exposure has not been identified to optimize bone formation over resorption. Preclinical studies showed that intermittent administration of PTH, as once daily subcutaneous injections, increases osteoblast recruitment, life span, and activity [2–5]. PTH also activates osteoclasts, and continuous exposure to PTH through intravenous infusion is accompanied by enough osteoclast stimulation that many of the benefits of intermittent exposure on bone remodeling become dampened [6,7]. When given daily instead of continuously, an increase in markers of bone formation precedes an increase in resorptive markers [8]. Hence, stimulation of resorption by PTH seems to lag behind stimulation of bone formation (Fig. 1).

There is a large body of preclinical studies of PTH and PTH fragments in the treatment and prevention of osteoporosis. A comprehensive review of these studies in animal models is beyond the scope of this article. To summarize, PTH therapy increases bone mass in healthy rats, prevents bone loss in newly estrogen-deficient rats, and increases bone mass in rodent and primate models of osteoporosis [9–14]. An important message from

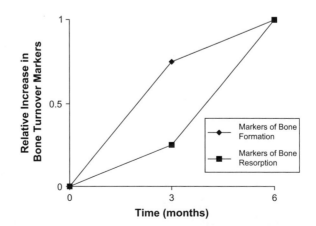

Fig. 1. Markers of bone turnover with daily subcutaneous PTH.

this preclinical work is that PTH seems to exert greater anabolic effect on trabecular than cortical bone formation.

Monotherapy for osteoporosis

Postmenopausal osteoporosis

The first landmark randomized double-blind placebo-controlled trial of rhPTH by Neer and colleagues [15] was published in 2001. In this phase III study, 1637 postmenopausal women who had pre-existing vertebral fractures were randomized to once daily injections of rhPTH (1-34), 20 μg or 40 μg, or placebo. All study subjects received 1000 mg of calcium and 200 to 1200 IU of vitamin D. The study was terminated early after a median follow-up of 21 months because of emerging data of an increased incidence of osteosarcomas in rats that were exposed to life-long high levels of rhPTH (1-34). The primary outcome in the trial by Neer and colleagues was the incidence of new vertebral fractures, which was 14% in the group that received placebo, compared with 5% and 4% in the groups that received 20 μg and 40 μg, respectively. The incidence of nonvertebral fractures was lower overall, but was statistically higher in the group that took placebo compared with the treatment groups (6% versus 3% in each of the treatment groups). Most nonvertebral fractures were categorized as wrist, rib, and "other," followed by humerus, hip, foot, ankle, and pelvic fractures. There was a dose response–related increase in BMD at the lumbar spine and femoral neck in each of the treatment groups; however, this was accompanied by a decrease in BMD of the radius. This finding prompted speculation that increases in trabecular BMD with PTH might be at the expense of cortical BMD, otherwise known as a "steal phenomenon"; however, analysis of cortical bone from iliac crest biopsies in a small subset of these subjects demonstrated increased cortical bone thickness in the treatment groups [16]. Because bone strength is a function of mineral content and cross-sectional area, most likely this small decrease in cortical BMD is not clinically significant. Moreover, the increase in cortical bone thickness may, in fact, confer greater overall bone strength. Based on the significant reduction in vertebral and nonvertebral fractures and the increases in BMD at the lumbar spine and femoral neck in postmenopausal women, the results of this study contributed significantly to FDA approval of teriparatide (rhPTH 1-34) in 2002.

Two important clinical trials investigated the efficacy of full-length rhPTH (1-84) on BMD and fracture risk in postmenopausal osteoporosis. The first, by Hodsman and colleagues [17], was a randomized double-blind placebo-controlled trial of 50 μg, 75 μg, or 100 μg of rhPTH (1-84) compared with placebo in 106 postmenopausal women who were not on other therapy for osteoporosis. After 12 months of follow-up the investigators demonstrated a dose-dependent increase in lumbar spine BMD compared with placebo (3.0%, 5.1%, and 7.7% increases in the treatment groups compared with 0.9% increase in the group that received placebo). Changes in BMD at the hip and femoral neck largely were nonsignificant. In a larger study, Ettinger and colleagues [18] randomized 2532 postmenopausal women who had osteoporosis to placebo or rhPTH (1-84), 100 μg daily. After 18 months, patients who were compliant with the study protocol had fewer new vertebral fractures (1.1% for rhPTH [1-84] versus 3.3% for placebo). In a subset of patients that had pre-existing vertebral fractures, the incidence of new vertebral fracture was 2.6% versus 8.4%, respectively. In all subjects, BMD at the spine, total hip, and femoral neck increased significantly with rhPTH (1-84) compared with placebo. To summarize, these two clinical trials of rhPTH (1-84) demonstrate dose-dependent improvements in trabecular and cortical BMD, the former to a greater extent. Preliminary fracture data are encouraging in the subsets of patients that had pre-existing vertebral fractures and in those who did not have fractures who were compliant with therapy [18].

Osteoporosis in men

Two studies reported increases in BMD in men who were given PTH, although fracture data are not yet available in this population. In the first trial, 437 men were randomized to rhPTH (1-34), 20 μg or 40 μg, or placebo [19]. All subjects had BMD T scores of the lumbar spine, femoral neck, or total hip that were less than or equal to -2.0 at baseline. After a median follow-up of 11 months, this trial also was halted prematurely because of the reported osteosarcomas in rat toxicity studies of rhPTH (1-34). The study groups each had increased lumbar spine and femoral neck BMD compared with the group that took placebo. The investigators also reported increased total body bone mineral content in each of the treatment groups. In a smaller study, 23 men who had osteoporosis, defined as a Z score of less than -2.0 or a T score of less than -2.5 at the lumbar spine or femoral neck, were randomized to 25 μg of a synthesized amino acid sequence of the hormone, hPTH (1-34) or placebo [20]. After 18 months, BMD at the lumbar spine and femoral neck increased significantly compared with placebo (13.5% and 2.9% increase at each site respectively). There was no increase in BMD at either site in the group that received placebo. Together, these studies suggest that the effect of PTH on BMD in men is similar to that in women; however, studies on fracture data are still necessary to understand fully the potential of PTH therapy in men.

Glucocorticoid-induced osteoporosis

The only randomized controlled trial of PTH for glucocorticoid-induced osteoporosis was in postmenopausal women on hormone replacement therapy with estrogen (HRT) [21]. In this study, 51 women who were taking at least 5 mg of daily prednisone and daily HRT were randomized to 25 μg of hPTH (1-34) daily plus HRT or HRT alone for 12 months. Lumbar spine

BMD increased 11.1% in the treatment group compared with no change in BMD in the control group. The change in total hip and femoral neck BMD was not significant after 12 months of treatment with PTH; however, Lane and colleagues [22] followed their cohort for another 12 months after completion of PTH therapy. They found that BMD of the total hip and femoral neck increased 4.7% ± 0.9% (P < .01) and 5.2% ± 1.3% respectively, compared to a small change of 1.3% ± 0.9% and 2.6% ± 1.7% in the control (estrogen-only) group. These results suggest that daily PTH increases BMD in the lumbar spine and hip in postmenopausal women who have glucocorticoid-induced osteoporosis who are taking HRT. They also suggest that the maximum anabolic effect on cortical bone mass at the hip may occur many months after PTH treatment is discontinued. As with studies in men, data on fracture outcomes for PTH in subjects who have glucocorticoid-induced osteoporosis have not yet emerged.

Combination therapy

Combination parathyroid hormone and bisphosphonates

In 2003, two landmark trials of PTH alone or in combination with bisphosphonates were published: one studied postmenopausal women who had osteoporosis or were at high risk for osteoporosis, and the other studied men with T scores of the lumbar spine or femoral neck of less than −2.0. The first study by Black and colleagues [23] randomized 238 postmenopausal women to rhPTH (1-84), 100 μg; alendronate, 10 mg; or combination therapy with both agents daily. After 12 months of follow-up, BMD increased at the lumbar spine in all three groups: 6.3% in the group that took PTH, 6.1% in the group that took combination therapy, and 4.6% in the group that took alendronate. Measurement of markers of bone turnover suggested that the ability of PTH to increase bone formation was dampened by concurrent administration of bisphosphonate therapy. BMD at the total hip and femoral neck remained unchanged in the group that took PTH, whereas it increased in the other groups. The use of quantitative CT demonstrated increased trabecular BMD of the lumbar spine in the group that took PTH, which was twice that of the other groups. In cortical bone, quantitative CT in the group that took PTH showed increases in volume, decreases in bone density, and no change in bone mineral content. The results of this study demonstrated no apparent additive benefit of PTH and bisphosphonates used in combination with respect to BMD at the lumbar spine, total hip, or femoral neck.

The second trial, by Finkelstein and colleagues [24], compared synthetic hPTH (1-34), 40 μg daily; alendronate, 10 mg daily; or both among 83 men with low BMD at baseline. The study duration was 30 months, and PTH was initiated after 6 months of bisphosphonate therapy alone in the group that received combination therapy. The group that took PTH had greater gains than did the other two groups in BMD at the lumbar spine and femoral neck. The group that received combination therapy had increased BMD at the lumbar spine compared with the group that took alendronate. Similar to the study by Black and colleagues, the results of this study showed no apparent additive benefit with combined treatment. In fact, bisphosphonate therapy seemed to attenuate increases in bone formation that were achieved with PTH alone.

The mechanism for this dampening of bone formation with the concurrent use of bisphosphonates is not clear; however, a clue may be found in the mechanism of PTH itself. PTH increases bone formation but also stimulates bone resorption through osteoblast production of receptor activator of NF-κB ligand (RANKL). Bone resorption, in turn, leads to the release of multiple growth factors (fibroblast growth factor [FGF-2], insulin-like growth factor [IGF-1], and transforming growth factor [TGF]-β) from the bone matrix. These growth factors stimulate osteoblast maturation and activity and augment angiogenesis (Fig. 2). Hurley and colleagues [25] demonstrated that knock-out mice for FGF-2 have a diminished anabolic response to PTH compared with normal controls. Because bisphosphonates inhibit bone resorption, the concurrent use of bisphosphonates with PTH in humans may impair the influence of these growth factors on increasing bone mass.

Sequential treatment (parathyroid hormone and bisphosphonates)

Preclinical studies of PTH demonstrated rapid increases in bone formation and gain in BMD that were lost quickly after discontinuation of therapy. The question arose as to whether gains in bone density with PTH could be maintained or enhanced with subsequent antiresorptive therapy. A small uncontrolled study by Rittmaster and colleagues [26] in 2000 measured BMD in 66 postmenopausal women who were assigned to daily rhPTH

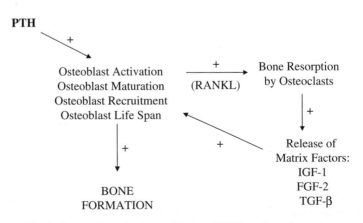

Fig. 2. Proposed mechanisms of action of PTH on bone formation.

(1-84), 50 µg, 75 µg, or 100 µg, or placebo for 1 year; all women received bisphosphonate for a subsequent year. Women who were assigned to 100 µg of rhPTH (1-84) followed by bisphosphonate had an impressive 14.6% increase in BMD at the lumbar spine. Increases at the total hip and femoral neck in the second year were more modest. Although the second year was neither a controlled nor blinded study, increases in BMD with sequential therapy were impressive and greater than other demonstrable treatment effects in previously published trials of estrogen or bisphosphonate therapy alone.

In a larger study, Black and colleagues [27] continued to study their cohort in a follow-up study of the combination trial with PTH and alendronate. Women who took PTH in the first-year trial were randomized to alendronate or placebo for an additional year. Women who took sequential PTH-alendronate experienced an increase in BMD at the spine and total hip (4.9% and 3.6%, respectively), whereas women who took sequential PTH-placebo experienced a decline in BMD of the spine (−1.7%) and no change in BMD of the hip. The investigators concluded that gains in BMD with PTH seem to be lost if not followed by subsequent bisphosphonate therapy. In fact, subsequent bisphosphonate therapy was associated with greater increases in BMD than was bisphosphonate therapy alone for the 2-year study duration.

Cyclic therapy (parathyroid hormone and bisphosphonates)

To capture the initial increases in bone formation without the subsequent enhanced bone resorption with long-term PTH therapy, Cosman and colleagues [28] studied the use of cyclic PTH in 126 women who had osteoporosis who already had been using bisphosphonates for approximately 3 years. Women were randomized to weekly alendronate, 70 mg; weekly alendronate plus synthetic hPTH (1-34), 25 µg daily; or weekly alendronate plus 3-month cycles on and off daily hPTH (1-34). There were no placebo injections, and the study was not blinded. Over 1 year of follow-up, markers of bone formation and resorption increased in both group that took PTH, but markers of resorption were lowest in the group that took cyclic PTH. This suggested that bone formation and resorption can be uncoupled with cyclic therapy. Increases in lumbar spine BMD were seen in both of the groups that took PTH, with no difference for cyclic or continuous daily PTH. Taking these and the results from the study by Black and colleagues into account, it remains to be determined if short cycles of PTH monotherapy followed by bisphosphonate will maximize the anabolic window of PTH and provide improvement in clinical outcomes (eg, fracture incidence).

Parathyroid hormone and estrogen or selective estrogen receptor modulator

Since the Women's Health Initiative reports of increased cardiovascular events and breast cancer in postmenopausal women who were on HRT, the use of HRT for osteoporosis has declined substantially. HRT should be reserved for the rare patient who cannot tolerate or has failed other modalities of treatment for osteoporosis and is willing to accept the small increases in absolute risk for these adverse events. Hence, combination therapy of PTH and HRT is worth mentioning only briefly. A 3-year study of synthetic hPTH (1-34) plus HRT versus HRT alone in 34 postmenopausal women who had been on HRT for at least 1 year demonstrated a 13.0% increase in BMD of the spine in the group that had combination therapy compared with no increase in the group that took HRT alone [8]. There were no placebo injections in the latter group, and the study was unblinded. Modest increases in total hip BMD (2.7%) and total body bone mineral content (8.0%) also were observed in the group that received combined treatment. Vertebral fractures (defined as a 15%–20% reduction in vertebral height on radiography) were reduced in the group that took combination therapy compared with the group that took HRT alone.

In a similar study, 52 women who had osteoporosis and who had been on HRT for at least 1 year were assigned to continued HRT or a combination of HRT and synthetic hPTH (1-34) for 3 years [29]. After 3 years, women who received combination therapy had 13%, 4%, and 4% increases in BMD at the spine, total hip, and total body, respectively, all of which were significantly greater than in the other group. In followup, BMD remained stable 1 year after discontinuation of PTH in the group that received combination therapy, which suggests that HRT alone could preserve the increased bone mass that was attributed to short-term PTH therapy. There also was a significant reduction in vertebral fractures in the group that received combination therapy, as measured by a 15% reduction in vertebral height.

In 2005, Deal and colleagues [30] presented a randomized clinical trial of rhPTH (1-34) alone or in combination with raloxifene for 6 months in 137 postmenopausal women who had osteoporosis (defined as T score of the spine, hip, or femoral neck of less than −2.5). There was no significant difference in increases in lumbar spine BMD between treatment groups. BMD of the total hip was significantly higher (2.2% increase) in the group that received combination therapy. Markers of bone formation were similar between groups, but markers of bone resorption were reduced by about 50% in the group that received combination therapy. These results are interesting in that they differ from trials of combined PTH and bisphosphonates; this suggests that the less "potent" antiresorptive agent raloxifene may be additive with respect to BMD gain when used with PTH. There is speculation that PTH and estrogen-like compounds may increase bone formation through modulation of similar Wnt signaling pathways, which may explain an additive effect. The trial was not designed to detect a difference in the incidence of vertebral or nonvertebral fractures.

Safety

In general, PTH has been tolerated well in clinical trials, and serious adverse events are rare (Table 2). In phase III trials the reported incidence of nausea and headache was up to 15% to 20% in patients who took rhPTH (1-34), 40 µg. In contrast, patients who took rhPTH (1-34), 20 µg, reported an incidence of headache and nausea that was comparable to placebo. Lightheadedness and fatigue also seem to be common in higher dosages. rhPTH (1-34) has only been approved for use as 20-µg daily injections; therefore, it is tolerated well. Local injection site reactions remain the most common side effect. Most frequently, local reactions are erythema or discomfort at the injection site. Rarely, patients develop subcutaneous nodules at the site of the injections, and these tend to resolve spontaneously after discontinuation of therapy. Initially, hypercalcemia or hypercalciuria was reported in up to 20% of patients who took higher dosages of rhPTH (1-34) (40 µg) and rhPTH (1-84) (100 µg). Hypercalcemia is less common (3%–7%) in patients who take lower (20 µg) dosages of rhPTH (1-34). The incidence of clinically significant hypercalcemia (serum calcium > 11.0 mg/dL or requiring reduction of the dosage or discontinuation of PTH) is low (1%–7%). Hypercalcemia peaks at 4 to 6 hours after PTH injection and generally returns to baseline within 24 hours of administration. Elevations in uric acid also have been reported in patients who take PTH, but a slightly higher incidence of gout in treatment subjects was reported in only one clinical trial. Creatinine clearance seems to increase in patients who take PTH, although the mechanism for this remains unclear.

Although there is concern over the development of osteosarcomas in rats that are given long-term PTH in toxicity studies, there have been no reported cases of osteosarcoma in the setting of PTH use in humans. In the toxicity studies, rats were given dosages of PTH that were 3 to 60 times higher than systemic exposure in humans who are given rhPTH (1-34), 20 µg daily. Osteosarcomas were observed at all toxic dosages and reached an incidence of 50% in the highest dosages. The risk for osteosarcoma in rats seems to be dependent on the dosage and duration of exposure to PTH [31]. There is no current evidence that PTH increases the risk for other malignancies. Women who took PTH in clinical trials occasionally developed newly diagnosed breast cancer. In each case, the development of breast cancer was deemed not to be related to PTH therapy. In Neer and colleagues' [15] phase III trial, more women who took placebo had a new diagnosis of cancer. Nonetheless, the safety of PTH therapy in women who have breast cancer or other malignancies has not been well established. PTH has not been studied in patients who have nephrolithiasis, although the rate of nephrolithiasis has not been shown to be greater in patients who take PTH.

Table 2
Summary of adverse events in clinical trials of parathyroid hormone

Investigators	Intervention	Physical side effects	Metabolic side effects	Drop-out rate
Neer et al	20 or 40 µg rhPTH (1-34) vs. placebo; 21 mo.	Nausea 18% (40 µg); HA 13% (40 µg); No difference in nausea or HA between 20-µg dosage and placebo.	Hypercalcemia 11% 40-µg dose and 3% 20-µg dosage[a]; Increased mean uric acid in PTH groups.	6% (20 µg)[a], 6% (40 µg), 11% (placebo).
Hodsman et al	50, 75, or 100 µg rhPTH (1-84) vs. placebo; 12 mo.	Nausea 24%, fatigue 16%.	Hypercalciuria 20%	12% (50 µg), 7% (75 µg), 22% (100 µg), 16% (placebo).
Ettinger et al	100 µg rhPTH (1-84) vs. placebo; 18 mo.	N/A	N/A	N/A
Orwoll et al	20 or 40 µg rhPTH (1-34) vs. placebo; 11 mo.	Nausea 18.7% (40 µg), HA 10.8% (40 µg).	N/A	9.3% (20 µg), 12.9% (40 µg), 4.8% (placebo).
Kurland et al	25 µg hPTH (1-34) vs. placebo; 18 months	N/A	Hypercalcemia in 20% on PTH	N/A
Lane et al	25 µg hPTH (1-34) vs. placebo; 12 mo. treatment, 24 months follow-up.	"Many" reported mild headaches	N/A	N/A
Black et al (year 1)	100 µg rhPTH (1-84) vs. combination with alendronate vs. alendronate alone; 12 mo.	No difference in nausea, HA, dizziness, or fatigue; increased uric acid in the PTH groups (including 3 women with gout).	Hypercalcemia in 12%, 14%, 0% PTH alone, combo, alendronate alone (required decrease in calcium supplements in some, reduction in PTH dose in 2 women).	No differences in drop-out rate

Finkelstein et al	40 µg hPTH 1-34 vs. combination with alendronate vs. alendronate alone; 30 mo.	Higher reported HA, dizziness, and musculoskeletal pain in the PTH groups	No significant difference in hypercalcemia; hypercalciuria 6% (PTH), 10.5% (combination), 2% (alendronate).	37% (PTH), 25% (combination), 11% (alendronate)
Rittmaster et al	50, 75, or 100 µg rhPTH (1-84) vs. placebo for 1 y followed by 1 y alendronate	N/A	N/A	N/A
Black et al (year 2)	Second year of alendronate vs. placebo	No difference in adverse events between groups (upper GI symptoms, HA, fatigue, nausea, injection reaction).	N/A	N/A
Cosman et al	25 µg daily vs. intermittent hPTH (1-34) combined with alendronate vs. alendronate alone; 12 mo.	More frequent musculoskeletal complaints in PTH groups (26% and 12%); erythema at injection site in PTH groups (3% and 18%).	1 in each PTH group with mildly elevated serum calcium; hypercalciuria 39% (daily PTH), 18% (cyclic PTH), 8% (alendronate).	12% (daily PTH), 15% (cyclic PTH), 16% (alendronate)
Lindsay et al	25 µg hPTH (-34) plus HRT vs. HRT alone; 3 y.	Frequently reported injection site reactions; few reports of SQ nodules.	N/A	24% (PTH + HRT); 0% (HRT alone).
Cosman et al	25 µg hPTH (1-34) plus HRT vs. HRT alone; 3 y.	No nausea; frequent injection site reactions; few SQ nodules.	No hypercalcemia	22% (PTH + HRT); 0% (HRT alone).
Deal et al	20 µg rhPTH (1-34) alone vs. rhPTH plus raloxifene; 6 mo.	Hot flashes 17.4% (PTH + raloxifene) 4.4% (PTH alone); vomiting 0% (PTH + raloxifene) 7.4% (PTH alone).	Hypercalcemia > 11 mg/dL 7% (PTH alone); 3% (PTH + raloxifene); increased uric acid in both groups.	17.4% (PTH + raloxifene); 11.8% (PTH alone).

Abbreviations: GI, gastrointestinal; HA, headache; hPTH, synthetic human parathyroid hormone; rhPTH, recombinant human parathyroid hormone; SQ, subcutaneous.

[a] Approved dosage.

Guidelines for use

rhPTH (1-34), 20 μg daily, is the only PTH formulation that is approved for use by the FDA, although an approval of rhPTH (1-84) is expected at the time of the writing of this article. Current indications and contraindications for use are listed in Box 1. PTH should be used in women who have osteoporosis who are at high risk for fracture and in men who have hypogonadal osteoporosis who are at high risk for fracture. A patient is considered to be at high risk for fracture if one or more of the following conditions are present: previous osteoporotic fractures, multiple risk factors for fracture, failure of previous therapy, and intolerance of previous therapy. Risk factors for fractures might include chronic secondary causes of osteoporosis, frail body habitus, family history of osteoporosis, or increased fall risk because of physical limitations. Occurrence of osteoporotic fractures while on therapy, worsening BMD despite therapy, or elevated markers of bone resorption on therapy are examples of treatment failures. These guidelines are supported by multiple well-designed controlled and uncontrolled clinical trials (Grade B). Recommended daily dosing is 20 μg rhPTH (1-34), although many studies of efficacy tested larger dosages of 40 μg daily. Most experts agree that PTH should be used for no more than 2 years, at least until longer-term safety studies are completed in human subjects. rhPTH (1-34), also known as teriparatide, is packaged as a 3-mL prefilled pen delivery device with an expiration of 28 days from the first injection; patients should be instructed to store pens in the refrigerator.

Box 1. Indications and contraindications for use of rhPTH (1-34)

Indications for use of rhPTH (1-34)
Women who have osteoporosis at high risk for fracture:
    Previous osteoporotic fracture
    Multiple risk factors for fracture
    Failure of previous therapy
    Intolerance to previous therapy

Men who have hypogonadal osteoporosis at high risk for fracture

Contraindications for use of rhPTH (1-34)
Hypercalcemia
Paget's disease of the bone
History of bone cancer
History of external radiation to the bone
Children
Pregnancy or nursing
Unexplained elevation in alkaline phosphatase

Future directions and unresolved issues

PTH increases BMD at the spine and hip in men and women who have osteoporosis, and reduces the incidence of vertebral and nonvertebral fractures in postmenopausal women who have osteoporosis. Further studies are needed to answer several questions, including whether there is a reduction in fracture incidence in men and if PTH can be administered safely for more than 2 years. Because PTH is an anabolic agent, its potential use in the setting of acute fracture healing is a potential area of interest. In addition, the use of PTH as preventive therapy in men and women who are at high risk for osteoporosis or in the setting of osteopenia has not been studied well. Because PTH is only available as subcutaneous injections, the inconvenience of administration precludes many patients from using it. Investigators are studying alternative application devices, including transdermal patches and intranasal and oral formulations. Lastly, as general clinical experience with PTH grows, more well-established safety in a broader range of comorbid conditions will be possible.

Summary

PTH is an exciting new treatment option for postmenopausal women and hypogonadal men who have osteoporosis. As an anabolic agent that affects bone metabolism, it represents an entirely new class of medication for osteoporosis and a novel approach to reducing fracture risk. Numerous clinical trials have demonstrated increases in trabecular and cortical BMD (trabecular more than cortical) in men and women, and reduction in vertebral and nonvertebral fractures in postmenopausal women. Studies suggest that it is safe for use for up to 2 years, but further studies are needed to test longer intervals of use. Although the combination of PTH and bisphosphonates does not seem to be additive, sequential therapy of PTH followed by bisphosphonate yields maximal gains in BMD compared with combined use or monotherapy with antiresorptive agents. As our knowledge of PTH grows, this is an exciting time for researchers, clinicians, and patients who study, treat, and live with the devastating consequences of progressive osteoporosis.

References

[1] United States Department of Health and Human Services. Bone health and osteoporosis: a report of the Surgeon General, 2004. Available at: http://www.surgeongeneral.gov/library/bonehealth/docs/exec_summ.pdf. Accessed on February 22, 2006.
[2] Dobnig H, Turner RT. Evidence that intermittent treatment with parathyroid hormone increases bone formation in adult rats by activation of bone lining cells. Endocrinology 1995; 136(8):3632–8.
[3] Leaffer D, Sweeney M, Kellerman LA, et al. Modulation of osteogenic cell ultrastructure by RS-23581, an analog of human parathyroid hormone (PTH)-related peptide-(1–34), and bovine PTH-(1–34). Endocrinology 1995;136(8):3624–31.

[4] Hodsman AB, Steer BM. Early histomorphometric changes in response to parathyroid hormone therapy in osteoporosis: evidence for de novo bone formation on quiescent cancellous surfaces. Bone 1993;14:523–7.

[5] Jilka RL, Weinstein RS, Bellido T, et al. Increased bone formation by prevention of osteoblast apoptosis with parathyroid hormone. J Clin Invest 1999;104:439–46.

[6] Dobnig H, Turner RT. The effects of programmed administration of human parathyroid hormone fragment (1–34) on bone histomorphometry and serum chemistry in rats. Endocrinology 1997;138(11):4607–12.

[7] Iida-Klein A, Lu SS, Kapadia R, et al. Short-term continuous infusion of human parathyroid hormone 1–34 fragment is catabolic with decreased trabecular connectivity density accompanied by hypercalcemia in C57BL/J6 mice. J Endocrinol 2005;186:549–57.

[8] Lindsay R, Nieves J, Formica C, et al. Randomised controlled study of effect of parathyroid hormone on vertebral-bone mass and fracture incidence among postmenopausal women on oestrogen with osteoporosis. Lancet 1997;350:550–5.

[9] Toromanoff A, Ammann P, Riond J-L. Early effects of short-term parathyroid hormone administration on bone mass, mineral content, and strength in female rats. Bone 1998;22:217–23.

[10] Hori M, Uzawa T, Morita K, et al. Effect of human parathyroid hormone (PTH(1–34)) on experimental osteopenia of rats induced by ovariectomy. Bone Miner 1988;3(3):193–9.

[11] Sato M, Zeng GQ, Turner CH. Biosynthetic human parathyroid hormone (1–34) effects on bone quality in aged ovariectomized rats. Endocrinology 1997;138(10):4330–7.

[12] Hock JM, Gera I, Fonseca J, et al. Human parathyroid hormone-(1–34) increases bone mass in ovariectomized and orchidectomized rats. Endocrinology 1988;122(6):2899–904.

[13] Oxlund H, Dalstra M, Ejersted C, et al. Parathyroid hormone induces formation of new cancellous bone with substantial mechanical strength at a site where it has disappeared in old rats. Eur J Endocrinol 2002;146:431–8.

[14] Brommage R, Hotchkiss CE, Lees CJ, et al. Daily treatment with human recombinant parathyroid hormone-(1–34), LY333334, for 1 year increases bone mass in ovariectomized monkeys. J Clin Endocrinol Metab 1999;84(10):3757–63.

[15] Neer RM, Arnaud CD, Zanchetta JR, et al. Effect of parathyroid hormone (1–34) on fractures and bone mineral density in postmenopausal women with osteoporosis. N Engl J Med 2001;344(19):1434–41.

[16] Jiang Y, Zhao JJ, Mitlak BH, et al. Recombinant human parathyroid hormone (1–34) [teriparatide] improves both cortical and cancellous bone structure. J Bone Miner Res 2003;18(11):1932–41.

[17] Hodsman AB, Hanley DA, Ettinger MP, et al. Efficacy and safety of human parathyroid hormone-(1–84) in increasing bone mineral density in postmenopausal osteoporosis. J Clin Endocrinol Metab 2003;88(11):5212–20.

[18] Ettinger MP, Greenspan SL, Barriott TB, et al. PTH (1–84) prevents first vertebral fracture in postmenopausal women with osteoporosis: results from the TOP study. Presented at the Annual Scientific Meeting of the American College of Rheumatology. San Antonio, October 21, 2004.

[19] Orwoll ES, Scheele WH, Paul S, et al. The effect of teriparatide [human parathyroid hormone (1–34)] therapy on bone density in men with osteoporosis. J Bone Miner Res 2003;18(1):9–17.

[20] Kurland ES, Cosman F, McMahon DJ, et al. Parathyroid hormone as a therapy for idiopathic osteoporosis in men: effects on bone mineral density and bone markers. J Clin Endocrinol Metab 2000;85(9):3069–76.

[21] Lane NE, Sanchez S, Modin GW, et al. Parathyroid hormone treatment can reverse corticosteroid-induced osteoporosis: results of a randomized controlled clinical trial. J Clin Invest 1998;102:1627–33.

[22] Lane NE, Sanchez S, Modin GW, et al. Bone mass continues to increase at the hip after para-thyroid hormone treatment is discontinued in glucocorticoid-induced osteoporosis: results of a randomized controlled clinical trial. J Bone Miner Res 2000;15(5):944–51.

[23] Black DM, Greenspan SL, Ensrud KE, et al. The effects of parathyroid hormone and alendr-onate alone or in combination in postmenopausal osteoporosis. N Engl J Med 2003;349(13): 1207–15.

[24] Finkelstein JS, Hayes A, Hunzelman JL, et al. The effects of parathyroid hormone, alendr-onate, or both in men with osteoporosis. N Engl J Med 2003;349(13):1216–26.

[25] Hurley MM, Okada Y, Xiao L, et al. Impaired bone anabolic response to parathyroid hor-mone in Fgf2$^{-/-}$ and Fgf2$^{+/-}$ mice. Biochem Biophys Res Commun 2006;341(4):989–94.

[26] Rittmaster RS, Bolognese M, Ettinger MP, et al. Enhancement of bone mass in osteoporotic women with parathyroid hormone followed by alendronate. J Clin Endocrinol Metab 2000; 85(6):2129–34.

[27] Black DM, Bilezikian JP, Ensrud KE, et al. One year of alendronate after one year of para-thyroid hormone (1–84) for osteoporosis. N Engl J Med 2005;353(6):555–65.

[28] Cosman F, Nieves J, Zion M, et al. Daily and cyclic parathyroid hormone in women receiv-ing alendronate. N Engl J Med 2005;353(6):566–75.

[29] Cosman F, Nieves J, Woelfert C, et al. Parathyroid hormone added to established hormone therapy: effects on vertebral fracture and maintenance of bone mass after parathyroid hor-mone withdrawal. J Bone Miner Res 2001;16(5):925–31.

[30] Deal C, Omizo M, Schwartz EN, et al. Combination teriparatide and raloxifene therapy for postmenopausal osteoporosis: results from a 6-month double-blind placebo-controlled trial. J Bone Miner Res 2005;20(11):1905–11.

[31] Eli Lilly and Company. Forteo® Package Insert PA 9242 FSAMP, 2004. Available at: http:// pi.lilly.com/us/forteo-pi.pdf. Accessed on March 22, 2006.

ELSEVIER
SAUNDERS

Rheum Dis Clin N Am 32 (2006) 721–731

RHEUMATIC
DISEASE CLINICS
OF NORTH AMERICA

Adherence to Medications for the Treatment of Osteoporosis

Stuart Silverman, MD

Department of Medicine, Division of Rheumatology, Cedars-Sinai Medical Center/UCLA,
The Osteoporosis Medical Center, 8641 Wilshire Boulevard, Suite 301,
Beverly Hills, CA 90211, USA

We now have a diverse menu of osteoporosis therapies, all of which significantly reduced the risk for fracture in randomized clinical trials; however, these encouraging results may not apply to patients who may not take their medications as prescribed. As the former Surgeon General C. Everett Koop once said, our medications only work when we take them. In the real world, the efficacy of therapies is limited by poor adherence. Therefore, it is important to understand why patients do not take their medications for osteoporosis.

Osteoporosis is a chronic, progressive asymptomatic illness that becomes symptomatic with fracture. Because osteoporosis is an asymptomatic illness for most patients, they may not be adherent because they do not understand how important it is to take their medication or how significant the benefits may be. Furthermore, improvements with their therapies are measured by changes in bone mineral density (BMD), which may take years.

This article discusses rates of adherence to medications in general, adherence to osteoporosis therapies, and the reasons that underlie poor adherence; it concludes by suggesting strategies to improve adherence.

Definitions

To understand the literature on adherence to osteoporosis medications, it is important to understand three words that often are used interchangeably, despite differences in meanings: compliance, persistence, and adherence. Compliance refers to how well a drug regimen is initiated and followed [1]. Compliance also includes taking the drug as prescribed by the clinician (eg,

---

E-mail address: stuarts@omcresearch.org

with water but not with milk, juice, or coffee). One way to measure compliance is to use the medication possession ratio (MPR) or the number of doses available to a patient over a fixed period of time; sometimes this is called refill compliance. For example, if a patient purchased an initial prescription for a bisphosphonate for 90 days and had one further 90-day refill over a 12-month period, then the MPR would equal approximately 180/360 or 50%. Persistence is the length of time that a patient takes a medication assuming no large refill gaps. Persistence on a medication may be expressed as the percentage of patients that is still on medication at a given time, such as 12 months with no gap in medication taking for a period of 30 days or more [2,3]. Adherence is a global term that encompasses compliance and persistence [4].

Measuring adherence

There are three main ways of measuring adherence: in clinical trials, by telephonic or mail survey, and by the use of observational databases. Each method has its own limitations. Subjects in clinical trials often have better adherence than do patients in the community [5]. Patients who are interviewed by telephone or by mail survey may overstate their adherence. Databases while more "real world" are also limited [4]. Initial prescription samples are not captured. When patients change insurance plans they may not be captured and may be believed to have discontinued medications. When studying adherence in a database it is important to have continuous enrollment in the health plan. Changes in a preferred drug may occur during the period of observation as well.

Adherence and chronic diseases

Patients have poor adherence to medication for chronic asymptomatic and chronic symptomatic illnesses [6]. Patients who have asymptomatic illnesses, such as hypertension or hyperlipidemias, take less than half of their prescribed medications [7]. This may be explained, in part, by the fact that these illnesses are silent. The absence of symptoms may make patients feel that medications are not necessary; however, even patients who have symptomatic illnesses (eg, congestive heart failure) still take only 70% of their medications [8]. It is estimated that 64% of hospital readmissions for heart failure are caused by nonadherence [9]. Claxton and colleagues [10] showed that, regardless of therapeutic area, mean adherence rates with all drugs were poor. Even a proportion of patients who have cancer display poor compliance; only about 80% take their medications as directed (range, 35%–97%).

Adherence with osteoporosis medications

Patients who have osteoporosis, like other patients who have chronic asymptomatic illnesses [11], often are noncompliant with their medication.

Studies have used self-report based on surveys as well as medical claims databases.

Using a telephone survey, Tosteson and colleagues [12] interviewed 956 women who had osteopenia or osteoporosis and who had been started on therapy. Approximately one quarter (19%–26%) of patients abandoned osteoporosis therapy within 7 months, regardless of the medication taken. More than two thirds of women who terminated therapy reported doing so because of side effects. Women who discontinued were more likely to do so because of side effects or uncertainty about the severity of their illness based on their bone density results; however, this study is limited in that it was based on self-report and may overestimate adherence.

Hamilton and colleagues [13] reported poor compliance with risedronate in clinical practice based on self-reported results from a questionnaire that was administered to patients who attended an osteoporosis clinic. A total of 219 patients was studied. Adverse events were reported by 38% of patients; they led to discontinuation of therapy in 19% of patients. Despite counseling by their health care providers and written instructions, 26% of all patients were not taking their osteoporosis medication correctly.

Medical claims databases have confirmed that patients who have osteoporosis have poor adherence to their therapies. McCombs and colleagues [14] looked at 58,000 patients (mostly female) in a large health insurance database who had started daily or weekly osteoporosis therapy. Persistence rates at 12 months were less than 25% for all therapies. The mean duration of therapy was low across all medications.

It was suggested that complex treatment regimens and dosing regimens, such as bisphosphonate therapy, may reduce the likelihood that patients will remain adherent to medication [6,10]. One solution may be to extend dosing intervals. Bisphosphonates are available with daily, weekly (alendronate, risedronate), and monthly (ibandronate) dosing regimens. Patients prefer extending dosing intervals for their bisphosphonate medications [15,16].

Ettinger and colleagues [17] examined persistence with daily and weekly bisphosphonate therapy in women who were older than 50 years of age by examining pharmacy claims from a longitudinal database that included approximately 25% of all retail pharmacies in the United States. Data were analyzed for new and continuing bisphosphonate users who received daily (n = 33,767) or weekly (n = 177,552) therapy. At 1 year, only 15.7% of new daily users and 31.4% of new weekly users were still on therapy. Among women who continued bisphosphonate treatment, 39.0% of patients who were taking daily bisphosphonates and 58.5% of weekly users remained on medication at the end of 1 year. All differences between persistence with daily versus weekly therapy were significant ($P < .0001$).

Using a pharmacy claims database of new users of oral bisphosphonate therapy and defining persistence as continuous therapy with no greater than a 45-day gap in medication coverage, Boccuzzi and colleagues [18] reported that only 18% of daily users and 22% of weekly users were persistent with treatment at 12 months.

Cramer and colleagues [2] used an administrative claims database from 30 health plans to identify 2741 women who were prescribed a daily or weekly bisphosphonate. After 12 months of therapy, only 31.7% and 44.2%, respectively, persisted on therapy. Patients who received weekly bisphosphonates obtained significantly more medication over the 12 months than did those who were prescribed daily bisphosphonates. Recker and colleagues [19], using a retail pharmacy database, found that only 25.2% of weekly and 13.2% of daily bisphosphonate users had adequate amounts of medication as defined by an MPR of more than 80%.

Adherence to osteoporosis medication in patients with glucocorticoid-induced osteoporosis

Curtis and colleagues [20] evaluated persistence and adherence to alendronate and risedronate among chronic glucocorticoid users who were enrolled in a United States managed care plan. Persistence was defined as no gap in medication for more than 180 days since the last bisphosphonate prescription. Despite adjustment for channeling (preferential prescribing of one medication over the other for patients who are at risk for gastrointestinal adverse events), no differences in adherence or persistence were noted between the two bisphosphonates. At 2 years, more than 50% of new users had discontinued bisphosphonate treatment. Factors that were associated with discontinuing therapy included advancing age, longer duration of bisphosphonate treatment, BMD test findings, and number of comorbidities.

Consequences of poor adherence to medications

Nonadherence to medication is the most significant reason why medications fail [2,21]. The consequences of nonadherence to medication depend on the disease and the characteristics of the medication. Patients who have asthma who are hospitalized or use emergency rooms frequently are more likely to be nonadherent to their medications [22]. In the CHARM (Candesartan in Heart Failure: Assessment of Reduction in Mortality and Morbidity) trials of candesartan in congestive heart failure, high adherence, even to placebo, was associated with lower mortality [23,24]. Outcomes, including decreased admissions to hospital for heart failure, were better in patients who were randomized to placebo who adhered to treatment (took their study medications more than 80% of the time) than in those who did not have high adherence (took their medications less than 80% of the time). Overall, the CHARM patients who were randomized to active medication had a 10% lower mortality than did patients who were randomized to placebo. Good adherence was associated with 35% decreased mortality in groups that took placebo and active medication. The investigators inter-preted this finding to suggest that adherence is a marker for adherence to effective treatments other than study medication, or to other adherence behaviors that affect outcomes. If correct, this explanation also may be germane to osteoporosis medications. Gold and Silverman [25] studied outcomes of the Choices self-management program and found significant correlations between adherence to one bone health behavior (eg, taking medication) and other behaviors (eg, exercise, taking calcium and vitamin D).

In a cohort of elderly patients (mean age, 76.6 years), it was estimated that 11.4% of drug-related hospital admissions were due to medication non-compliance. Further, approximately one quarter of total hospital costs for drug-related admissions were linked to noncompliance [24].

Consequences of poor adherence to osteoporosis medications

Poor adherence to osteoporosis medications has been associated with less improvement in BMD, less suppression of bone turnover markers, and in-creased risk for fractures. Yood and colleagues [26] studied the relationship between compliance to osteoporosis medication and changes in BMD in pa-tients who were initiating therapy. Compliance was defined as the percent of time that patients refilled their prescriptions and BMD values were obtained at study end (mean follow-up, 590 days). Among participants with refill compliance of at least 66%, mean increases in spine BMD were 3.8% per year; patients with refill compliance of up to 66% had mean increases in BMD of 2.1% per year. Clowes and colleagues [27] studied the relationship between adherence and BMD and bone turnover markers (urinary N-telo-peptide of type I collagen [uNTX], a marker of bone resorption). In this study, cumulative adherence was calculated as number of tablets taken/ number of tablets prescribed since randomization, using an electronic mon-itoring device. Adherence to therapy at 1 year was correlated positively to percent changes in hip BMD ($P = .01$, but not lumbar spine BMD) and suppression of uNTX ($P = .002$) from baseline.

A more important consequence of poor adherence is increased fracture risk. Caro and colleagues [28] studied the relationship between adherence and fracture risk using a claims database of 11,000 women in Saskatchewan, Canada. Compliance was defined as an MPR of 0.80 (drug available 80% of the time). Compliant patients experienced a 16% lower fracture rate compared with noncompliant patients (hazard ratio, 0.81; $P = .0009$).

Siris and colleagues [29] did a retrospective analysis of claims made for bisphosphonate therapy during a 5-year period (1/1/1999–12/31/2003) using two large pharmaceutical databases. The eligible cohort included 35,537 women who were at least 45 years of age, prescribed a bisphosphonate, with data available for a 24-month period after the index prescription. Per-sistence was defined as no gap in refills for more than 30 days over 24 months, and refill compliance was defined as an MPR of at least 80%.

Forty-three percent of women were refill compliant and 20% were persistent with bisphosphonate therapy over the 24-month study period. Women who achieved compliance with therapy had a 21% reduction in fractures overall compared with those who were not compliant. The adjusted relative risk for all nonvertebral fractures was 20% lower in women who were refill compliant compared with those who were not ($P < .0001$). When hip fractures were analyzed separately, the adjusted risk was 37% lower for compliant women ($P < .0001$ versus noncompliant women). Wrist fractures were less common in compliant women, but this difference was not statistically significant. There was a progressive relationship between refill compliance and fracture risk reduction that was first evident at refill compliance rates around 50%, but it became more evident as compliance rates increased to at least 75%.

McCombs and colleagues [14] also used a large medical claims database. They found that good compliance with therapy was associated with decreased fracture risk and decreased health care costs. Compliance in this database analysis reduced the risk for hip fracture (odds ratio [OR], 0.382; $P < .01$) and vertebral fracture (OR, 0.601; $P < .05$). Further, compliant patients used fewer physician services, fewer hospital outpatient services, and less hospital care.

Barriers to adherence to medication

Factors that are associated with poor adherence include age, socioeconomic status (education, income, occupation, and population density), complexity of medical regimens, and social support and participation [30]. The relationship between adherence and social activities may represent higher motivation to adhere to treatment in those who are engaged in more enjoyable activities or individuals who are less isolated or depressed [31]. Adherence also is influenced strongly by the community in which patients live, how health providers practice medicine in that community, and the type of medical provider. The presence of psychiatric conditions, particularly depression, can impede adherence to medication regimens. In addition, cognitive impairment or dementia has a negative effect on adherence. Asymptomatic diseases, negative side effects, and complexity of treatment regimens impact adherence. Finally, inadequate follow-up on the part of the physician or other health care professional or poor discharge planning can lead to poor adherence rates [6].

The health belief model may be helpful in understanding additional barriers to adherence. Patients who lack insight into their illness and into the consequences of their illness and poor adherence to medication regimens are less likely to take their medications [25]. Similarly, patients who do not believe that treatment will be beneficial are less likely to be adherent. Finally, missed office appointments can be a sign of poor adherence and should be followed up [6].

Why is adherence with osteoporosis medications so poor?

A variety of factors may be involved directly or indirectly in poor adherence to osteoporosis medications. These include inadequate information about osteoporosis and the medication, concerns about drug-associated adverse effects, costs, and problems that are associated with treating older patients.

Patients may not understand their diagnosis of osteoporosis or their medication. Pickney and Arnason [32] studied the relationship between understanding of dual-energy x-ray absorptiometry (DXA) results and adherence. The investigators queried 1000 residents of rural Wisconsin who had had a DXA test. Only 63% of those with normal BMD correctly recalled this; only 31% of patients who had osteopenia and 50% of patients who had osteoporosis correctly remembered their results. Patients who had had a low BMD and who remembered their results as being low were significantly more likely to continue taking their osteoporosis medication. This finding emphasizes the importance of good communication with patients and patient understanding of their diagnosis. Correct understanding of DXA information may lead to improved adherence in patients with low BMD.

In a recent survey, more than half (51%) of women who were prescribed osteoporosis medication did not recall how long they were to take it [33]. A few women believed that they only needed to remain on therapy for 6 months or until their present course was finished. In this same survey, 27% of women believed that their risk for fracture was the same, regardless of whether they took their osteoporosis medication. Twenty percent were unaware of treatment benefits, and 17% did not believe that their treatment had any benefit at all. Side effects and restrictions on how to take medications were the main drawbacks that were associated with treatment in the survey; staying upright was the biggest inconvenience associated with bisphosphonate therapy.

Often, patients who have osteoporosis are elderly. The elderly frequently have concurrent illnesses and conditions that require multiple medications, along with some degree of memory loss. Roth and Ivey [34] evaluated 100 elderly patients in the community who took an average of 9.6 medications; nonadherence was high at 53%.

Two recent studies looked at factors that influence adherence. Papaioannou and colleagues [35] in Canada found that two factors—prevalent vertebral fracture and older age—predicted better adherence. Solomon and colleagues [36], using a managed care claims database, found that female gender, younger age, multiple medications, multiple comorbid conditions, prevalent fracture, and nursing home residency also predicted adherence.

Strategies for improving adherence to osteoporosis medications

A variety of strategies to encourage better adherence to therapies has been proposed; however, a recent Cochrane review found that less than half of interventions tested in randomized trials improved adherence and less than one third improved outcomes [37] Effective interventions usually were complex and involved combinations of several interventions, not simply one intervention. Interventions did not have sustained benefits beyond 6 months. It is not known which of the multiple components of these interventions were the most effective [37]. Integrating patient preferences into treatment plans may be the most practical way to improve adherence [38].

One strategy may be to use osteoporosis medications with extended dosing intervals. The development of medications, such as oral bisphosphonates that are administered once monthly (ibandronate), intravenous bisphosphonates that are administered every 3 months (ibandronate), or agents that are injected subcutaneously twice yearly (denosumab) or infused once yearly (zoledronate) may provide an opportunity to improve adherence. The use of medications with extended dosing intervals may increase the likelihood of forgetting medications, however, with associated greater clinical consequences.

The use of patient reminder programs may be extremely important for reinforcing treatment adherence, especially with extended dosing intervals. Patient reminder programs use telephone or ordinary mail. Newer techniques, such as cell phone reminders, medication kits with paging systems, or e-mail are being evaluated. A current patient reminder program found that up to 66% of individuals who had osteoporosis preferred e-mail as a reminder system.

Confirmation of improved adherence with extended dosing intervals will rely on data from medical claims databases. It is not known whether there is a maximum adherence that can be achieved simply by extending dosing intervals.

It has been assumed that giving feedback to patients would improve adherence. Such information could be bone marker or BMD information. Because most patients may stop their osteoporosis medication before 1 or 2 years when bone density is assessed, there has been interest in studying the impact of bone turnover information.

The author's group studied the use of bone turnover marker information to improve compliance. Nattras and colleagues [39] randomized 280 patients to four study arms: uNTX levels at 3 months, patient education, uNTX levels and patient education, and no intervention. After 12 months no differences were seen in the number of months on therapy between these four groups. All patients were seen by a health care provider at 3 months. A visit with a health care provider at 3 months may be more important reinforcement than the bone marker information.

In a study by Clowes and colleagues [27], patients who were monitored by a nurse had greater adherence to osteoporosis therapy than did those who received no monitoring. Patients who met with a nurse had equivalent adherence to those who met with a nurse and received bone marker information. In a third study on bone marker information, 2302 postmenopausal women, aged 65 to 80 years, who had osteoporosis were studied in a 1-year multicenter study [40]. Persistence was measured by an electronic sensing device in the medication bottle. Trial sites were randomized into two groups: reinforcement groups that received bone marker information at weeks 10 and 22 and groups that did not receive bone marker information. There was 13% less persistence in groups that did not receive bone marker information (hazards ratio = 0.87; P = .16); however, the overall persistence rates were surprisingly high for both study groups (79.8% and 77.2%). Therefore, these three studies did not show significant effects of bone marker information as feedback to improve adherence.

For rheumatologists to improve adherence to osteoporosis or other rheumatic disease therapies, they need to form a partnership with their patients that is based on communication and trust. Patients need to understand that they have osteoporosis and that osteoporosis is associated with significant negative consequences (eg, fracture with increased morbidity and mortality and decreased quality of life). Patients also need to understand that there are medications that can reduce their risk for fracture. Rheumatologists need to talk with their patients about their concerns about these medications and their side effects; about barriers to taking these medications and how to resolve these barriers; and about their preferences for dosing interval. These preferences may be based on their lifestyles and needs. Listening to these preferences may improve adherence and improve outcomes.

Summary

Although there is a wide variety of osteoporosis medications with varying dosing intervals, adherence to therapies for postmenopausal- or glucocorticoid-induced osteoporosis remains poor. It is associated with long-term consequences, such as increased osteoporotic fractures, including nonvertebral and hip fractures. There is a lack of understanding about why patients are not staying on therapy. Potential solutions include newer medications with extended dosing intervals, monitoring, and an open physician–patient relationship.

References

[1] Sclar DA, Chin A, Skaer TL, et al. Effect of health education in promoting prescription refill compliance among patients with hypertension. Clin Ther 1991;13(4):489–95.
[2] Cramer JA, Amonkar MM, Hebborn A, et al. Compliance and persistence with bisphosphonate dosing regimens among women with postmenopausal osteoporosis. Curr Med Res Opin 2005;21(9):1453–60.
[3] Sikka R, Xia F, Aubert RE. Estimating medication persistency using administrative claims data. Am J Manag Care 2005;11(7):449–57.
[4] Dezii CM. Persistence with drug therapy: a practical approach using administrative claims data. Manag Care 2001;10(2):42–5.

[5] Hart JT. Commentary: can health outputs of routine practice approach those of clinical trials? Int J Epidemiol 2001;30(6):1263–7.

[6] Osterberg L, Blaschke T. Adherence to medication. N Engl J Med 2005;353(5):487–97.

[7] Benner JS, Glynn RJ, Mogun H, et al. Long-term persistence in use of statin therapy in elderly patients. JAMA 2002;188:455–61.

[8] Roe CM, Motherall BR, Teitelbaum F, et al. Angiotensin-converting enzyme inhibitor compliance and dosing among patients with heart failure. Am Heart J 1999;138:818–25.

[9] Ghali JK, Kadakia S, Cooper R, et al. Precipitating factors leading to decompensation of heart failure: traits among urban blacks. Arch Intern Med 1988;148:2013–6.

[10] Claxton AJ, Cramer J, Pierce C. A systematic review of the associations between dose regimens and medication compliance. Clin Ther 2001;23(8):1296–310.

[11] Miller NH. Compliance with treatment regimens in chronic asymptomatic diseases. Am J Med 1997;102(2A):43–9.

[12] Tosteson AN, Grove MR, Hammond CS, et al. Early discontinuation of treatment for osteoporosis. Am J Med 2003;115(3):209–16.

[13] Hamilton B, McCoy K, Taggart H. Tolerability and compliance with risedronate in clinical practice. Osteoporos Int 2003;14(3):259–62.

[14] McCombs JS, Thiebaud P, McLaughlin-Miley C, et al. Compliance with drug therapies for the treatment and prevention of osteoporosis. Maturitas 2004;48(3):271–87.

[15] Simon JA, Lewiecki EM, Smith ME, et al. Patient preference for once weekly alendronate 70 mg versus once daily alendronate 10 mg: a multicenter randomized open label crossover study. Clin Ther 2002;24:1871–86.

[16] Simon JA, Beusterien K, Leidy NK, et al. Women with postmenopausal osteoporosis express a preference for once-monthly versus once-weekly bisphosphonate treatment. Female Patient 2005;30:31–6.

[17] Ettinger M, Gallagher R, Amonkar M, et al. Medication persistence is improved with less frequent dosing of bisphosphonates, but remains inadequate. Arthritis Rheum 2004;50:S513.

[18] Boccuzzi SF, Omar SH, Kahler MA, et al. Assessment of adherence and persistence with daily and weekly dosing regimens of oral bisphosphonates. Presented at the European Congress on Clinical and Economic Aspects of Osteoporosis and Osteoarthritis (ECCEO), Rome, Italy. March 16–19, 2005.

[19] Recker RR, Gallagher R, Mac Cosbe PE. Effect of dosing frequency on bisphosphonate medication adherence in a large longitudinal cohort of women. Mayo Clin Proc 2005;80: 856–61.

[20] Curtis JR, Westfall AO, Allison JJ, et al. Persistence and adherence to alendronate and risedronate among chronic glucocorticoid users [abstract]. Arthritis Rheum 2005;52(9 Suppl): s374.

[21] O'Brien MK, Petrie K, Raeburn J. Adherence to medication regimens: updating a complex medical issue. Med Care Rev 1992;49(4):435–54.

[22] Bender B, Milgrom H, Rand C. Nonadherence in asthmatic patients: is there a solution to the problem? Ann Allergy Asthma Immunol 1997;79(3):177–85 [quiz 185–6].

[23] Granger BB, Swedberg K, Ekman I, et al, for the CHARM investigators. Adherence to candesartan and placebo and outcomes in congestive heart failure in the CHARM programme: double blind, randomized controlled trial. Lancet 2005;366:2005–11.

[24] Col N, Fanale JE, Kronholm P. The role of medication noncompliance and adverse drug reactions in hospitalizations of the elderly. Arch Intern Med 1990;150(4):841–5.

[25] Gold DT, Silverman SL. Osteoporosis self-management: Choices For Better Bone Health. South Med J 2004;97(6):551–4.

[26] Yood RA, Emani S, Reed JI, et al. Compliance with pharmacologic therapy for osteoporosis. Osteoporos Int 2003;14(12):965–8.

[27] Clowes JA, Peel NF, Eastell R. The impact of monitoring on adherence and persistence with antiresorptive treatment for postmenopausal osteoporosis: a randomized controlled trial. J Clin Endocrinol Metab 2004;89(3):1117–23.

[28] Caro JJ, Ishak KJ, Huybrechts KF, et al. The impact of compliance with osteoporosis therapy on fracture rates in actual practice. Osteoporos Int 2004;15(12):1003–8.

[29] Siris E, Harris ST, Rosen C, et al. Adherence to bisphosphonate therapy and fracture rates in osteoporotic women. Relationship to vertebral and non-vertebral fractures from a US claims database. Mayo Clin Proc 2006;81(8):1013–22.

[30] McDonald K, Ledwidge M, Cahill J, et al. Elimination of early rehospitalization in a randomised, controlled trial of multidisciplinary care in a high risk elderly heart failure population. Eur J Heart Fail 2001;3:209–15.

[31] Irvine J, Baker B, Smith J, et al. Poor adherence to placebo or amiodarone therapy predicts mortality: results from the CAMIAT study. Psychosom Med 1999;61:566–75.

[32] Pickney CS, Arnason JA. Correlation between patient recall of bone densitometry results and subsequent treatment adherence. Osteoporos Int 2005;16(9):1156–60.

[33] IPSOS Health. European Survey of Physicians and Women with Osteoporosis. Sponsored by Roche-GSK. January April 2005.

[34] Roth MT, Ivey JL. Self reported medication use in community residing older adults: a pilot study. Am J Geriat Pharmacother 2005;3:196–204.

[35] Papaioannou A, Ioannidis G, Adachi JD, et al. Adherence to bisphosphonates and hormone replacement therapy in a tertiary care setting of patients in the CANDOO database. Osteoporos Int 2003;14(10):808 13.

[36] Solomon DH, Avorn J, Katz JN, et al. Compliance with osteoporosis medications. Arch Intern Med 2005;165(20):2414–9.

[37] Haynes RB, Yao X, Degani A, et al. Interventions to enhance medication adherence. Cochrane Database Syst Rev 2005;4:CD000011.

[38] Bissell P, May CR, Noyce PR. From compliance to concordance: barriers to accomplishing a re-framed model of health care interactions. Soc Sci Med 2004;58:851–62.

[39] Nattras S, Silverman S, Drinkwater B. Effectiveness of education and/or NTx results as a means of encouraging compliance to alendronate. Presented at World Congress on Osteoporosis, Chicago, Illinois. June 15–18, 2000

[40] Delmas PD, Vrijens B, Roux C, et al. Reinforcement message based on bone turnover marker response influences long-term persistence with risedronate in osteoporosis: The IMPACT Study. J Bone Miner Res 2003;18(Suppl 2):S374.

RHEUMATIC
DISEASE CLINICS
OF NORTH AMERICA

Rheum Dis Clin N Am 32 (2006) 733–757

Glucocorticoid-Induced Osteoporosis: Mechanisms and Therapeutic Approach

Jean-Pierre Devogelaer, MD

*Department of Medicine, Arthritis Unit, Saint-Luc University Hospital,
Université catholique de Louvain, 10, Avenue Hippocrate, UCL 5390,
B-1200 Brussels, Belgium*

Glucocorticoids (GCs) are among the most universally prescribed drugs, owing to their immunosuppressive and anti-inflammatory potency. Their therapeutic activity is of utmost importance in conditions treated by various medical specialists, such as rheumatologists, hematologists, allergologists, internists, pneumologists, dermatologists. When compound E (cortisone) became available nearly 60 years ago, enthusiasm about its favorable action on stiffness, pain, and joint inflammation in rheumatic conditions [1] was rapidly followed by adverse reports of hypercortisolism [1,2]. In unconsidered use, the beneficial effects of GCs are more than counterbalanced by side effects such as cataracts, skin atrophy, truncal obesity, fluid retention, myopathy, and glucose and lipid disturbances. Even careful use is not completely free of after-effects. One of the most conspicuous complications of GC therapy is osteoporosis (OP), with its host of fractures that may occur soon after the initiation of GC therapy. GC-OP is by far the most frequent cause of secondary OP, as is exemplified in a recent meta-analysis [3]. In this study, totaling approximately 42,000 men and women, the relative risk for OP fracture in general ranged from 2.63 to 1.71, and the specific risk for hip fracture ranged from 4.42 to 2.48, respectively, at the ages of 50 and 85 years [3]. The fracture risk was similar in men and women, independent of prior fracture, and was only partially explained by bone mineral density (BMD) [3]. In a retrospective study of a large cohort of 244,235 oral GC users compared with the same number of controls (58.6% being women), a relative incidence of 1.61 for hip fracture and of 2.60 for vertebral fracture was observed [4]. The risk was commensurate to the daily dose, with no truly safe dose (Table 1). Moreover, all fracture risks decreased rapidly after cessation of oral GC therapy, suggesting reversibility of the risks [4].

E-mail addresses: devogelaer@ruma.ucl.ac.be; jean-pierre.devogelaer@uclouvain.be

Table 1
Fracture risk according to dose of oral glucocorticoids (N = 244,235)

	Low dose (n = 50,649)		Medium dose (n = 104,833)		High dose (n = 87,949)	
	No. of cases	Adjusted relative rate (95% CI)	No. of cases	Adjusted relative rate (95% CI)	No. of cases	Adjusted relative rate (95% CI)
Nonvertebral	2192	1.17 (1.10–1.25)	2486	1.36 (1.28–1.43)	1665	1.64 (1.54–1.76)
Forearm	531	1.10 (0.96–1.25)	526	1.04 (0.93–1.17)	273	1.19 (1.02–1.39)
Hip	236	0.99 (0.82–1.20)	494	1.77 (1.55–2.02)	328	2.27 (1.94–2.66)
Vertebral	191	1.55 (1.20–2.01)	440	2.59 (2.16–3.10)	400	5.18 (4.25–6.31)
		≤ 2.5 mg/d		2.5–7.5 mg/d		≥ 7.5 mg/d

Abbreviation: CI, confidence interval.
From Van Staa TP, LeuFkens HGM, Abenhaim L, et al. Use of oral corticosteroids and risk of fractures. J Bone Miner Res 2000;15(6):993–1000; with permission of the American Society for Bone and Mineral Research.

The frequency of the complication and its rapid occurrence should justify systematic preventive measures. In a recent paper, only approximately 40% of patients taking oral GCs had undergone some form of bone mass measurement or had received some prescription medications to prevent or treat OP [5]. However, the frequency of bone mass measurements had increased threefold and the use of prescription medications twofold compared with the conditions observed 5 to 6 years before [5]. These numbers remain, unfortunately, too low, despite an encouraging upward temporal trend. Increases in the relative risks for fracture have also been observed in children [6]. The mechanisms leading to an increase in bone fragility are not completely understood. It is an universal observation that bone loss and fragility are more marked at skeletal sites with more trabecular bone (eg, ribs and vertebral bodies) [7–10]. Nonetheless, BMD of the upper extremity of the femur, mostly composed of cortical bone, is also subject to bone loss [10].

Glucocorticoid preparations and modes of administration

Cortisol or hydrocortisone is naturally secreted by the adrenal glands. Its excess in Cushing's syndrome has been known for more than 60 years to provoke diminished bone mass [11]. Synthetic derivatives have been synthesized with the aim of decreasing the frequency of side effects of hydrocortisone, while maintaining (or even increasing) its therapeutic activity. For example, a double bond introduced in position 1 to 2 as for prednisone, prednisolone led to a fourfold increase in anti-inflammatory potency (Table 2). Cortisone must be converted to cortisol and prednisone to prednisolone to become biologically active. Acquisition of metabolic activity requires the action of the enzyme 11 β-hydroxysteroid dehydrogenase type 1,

Table 2
Some glucocorticoid preparations

	Respective potencies		
	Anti-inflammatory	Equivalence (mg)	Sodium retaining
With a biologic half-life <12 hours			
Hydrocortisone	1	20	++
Cortisone	0.8	25	++
With a biologic half-life between 12 and 36 hours			
Prednisone	4	5	+
Prednisolone	4	5	+
Methylprednisolone	5	4	0
Triamcinolone	5	4	0
Deflazacort	4	6	0
With a biologic half-life >48 hours			
Paramethasone	10	2	0
Betamethasone	25	0.60	0
Dexamethasone	30	0.75	0

which increases with age and glucocorticoid exposure [12]. However, 11 β-hydroxysteroid dehydrogenase type 2 inactivates the conversion of cortisol and prednisolone to cortisone and prednisone, respectively. These metabolic steps could have some involvement in the development of toxicity. Unfortunately, it is not evident that bone loss has been reduced with the use of the synthetic derivatives, perhaps with the exception of the oxazoline derivative of prednisone (deflazacort) [13,14] However, the generally admitted anti inflammatory equipotency of deflazacort (6 mg) versus prednisone (5 mg) [15] has been questioned ever since [16]. It should be recalled that the bioequivalences provided in Table 2 are mean values and not definite face values blindly applicable to individual cases. Because GCs are most frequently administered orally, oral administration has been studied the most, as far as bone metabolism is concerned. Other types of administration, such as inhaled [17] and topical GCs, may also have some detrimental effect on BMD, with the remarkable exception of high-dose short-term GC therapy [18], even if bone turnover markers are transiently modified [19].

Pathophysiology

The pathophysiology of GC-OP is not yet completely understood. Numerous factors have been incriminated in the occurrence of OP after GC use. Both daily dose and treatment duration, therefore cumulative dose, have been considered responsible for the skeletal adverse effects of GCs. However, because fractures in GC users occur rapidly after initiation of GCs, these adverse effects appear to be essentially related to daily dose rather than to duration of therapy or cumulative dose [3,4,20]. Indeed, fractures occur in GC-OP at a higher BMD than in postmenopausal OP [3,21]. This consideration pleads in favor of rapid institution of preventive measures. Moreover, patients prescribed GCs are frequently suffering from systemic diseases, such as rheumatoid arthritis, that could constitute a risk factor for low BMD [22].

Gender and age

Age, gender, and menopausal status play a role in the development of GC-OP. In children, GCs slow down bone modeling and remodeling. They impair linear growth and provoke bone loss by several mechanisms: decrease in intestinal calcium absorption; interference with the growth hormone-insulin growth factor 1 axis; inhibition of chondrocyte proliferation, proteoglycan synthesis, and osteoblast recruitment and function; and increase in apoptosis of hypertrophic chondrocytes [23–26]. In adults, a greater bone loss is seen in patients older than 50 years (postmenopausal females and males) [27]. At doses less than and equal to 7.5 mg/d prednisolone, GCs do not provoke significant bone loss at the forearm [8], at the lumbar spine [28,29], and at the hip [29] in premenopausal women, in contrast with men and postmenopausal women [8]. Higher doses of GCs have a deleterious effect on BMD whatever the gender or the menopausal status (Fig. 1) [28–32]. In a prospective study, at a mean starting dose of 18 mg prednisolone per day, the incidence of morphometric vertebral fractures amounted after 1 year to 0% in premenopausal women (mean age 41.5 years), 16% in postmenopausal women (mean age 64.2 years), and 24% in men (mean age 54.9 years) in the placebo group (Fig. 2) [29,30,32]. At these mean ages, the figures correspond to a dramatic increase in fracture risk over those who do not use GCs.

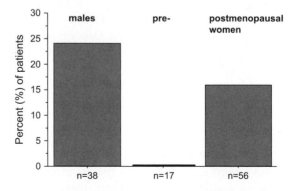

Fig. 1. Incidence (percentage) of vertebral fractures in patients on glucocorticoids (mean starting dose: 18 mg/d) and receiving placebo for 1 year. (*Adapted from* Reid DM, Adami S, Devogelaer J-P, et al. Risedronate increases bone density and reduces vertebral fracture risk within one year in men on corticosteroid therapy. Calcif Tissue Int 2001;69(4):242–7; with kind permission of Springer Science and Business Media.).

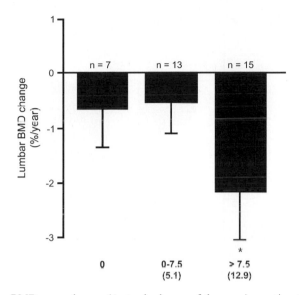

Fig. 2. Lumbar BMD mean changes (+ standard error of the mean) over time (percentage per year) in premenopausal women according to the prednisolone daily dose in milligrams (mean), followed up for 21 months. There was no statistical difference between the three subgroups regarding age, body mass index, or baseline BMD. (*From* Jardinet D, Lefèbvre C, Depresseux G, et al. Longitudinal analysis of bone mineral density in pre-menopausal female systemic lupus erythematosus patients: deleterious role of glucocorticoid therapy at the lumbar spine. Rheumatology 2000;39(4):389–92; with permission.)

Bone metabolism

GCs provoke a dramatic decrease in bone formation and an increase in bone resorption, the latter being less pronounced [33]. Bone loss develops rapidly after institution of therapy and involves preferably the trabecular compartment of the skeleton (see Fig. 2) [7–9,28–32]. The bone loss is more marked during the first months of therapy and slows down thereafter. This pattern is exemplified in Fig. 3 [28,30–32]. Patients who had the higher cumulative GC dose (ie, those treated for a longer period) lost BMD at a lower rate than patients who had started GC therapy more recently [28] and therefore received a lower cumulative GC dose. Several factors may contribute to the changes in bone metabolism induced by GCs (Fig. 4). In addition to the various illustrated factors that potentially act in isolation or synergistically, others could help to explain the individual difference in sensitivity and in severity of after-effects of GCs: the variability in absorption of the orally administered hormone, the distribution in the body and the clearance of prednisolone in the liver [34], the number and the specificity of the GC receptors [35], the activity of the enzyme 11 β-hydroxysteroid dehydrogenase type 1 expressed in osteoblasts and increasing with aging [12], and a low BMD before GC therapy. Some patients have their skeletons

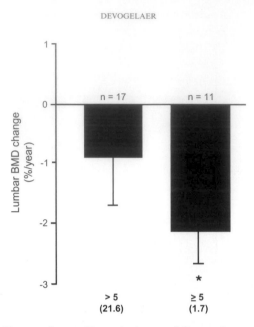

Fig. 3. Lumbar BMD mean changes (± standard error of the mean) over time (percentage per year) in premenopausal women according to the cumulative GC doses in grams (mean) at baseline. The patients who had received the higher GC cumulative doses had a lower annual loss in lumbar BMD than the patients who had received a lower GC dose. (*From* Jardinet D, Lefèbvre C, Depresseux G, et al. Longitudinal analysis of bone mineral density in pre-menopausal female systemic lupus erythematosus patients: deleterious role of glucocorticoid therapy at the lumbar spine. Rheumatology 2000;39(4):389–92; with permission.)

relatively spared in spite of high GC doses, and others present with patent complications with small doses.

The understanding of the mechanisms may be of some clinical relevance, because they have some implications for the indication of preventive or curative therapy for GC-OP. GCs provoke a small increase in bone resorption, which could be explained by some degree of secondary hyperparathyroidism [36,37]. The secondary hyperparathyroidism is believed to develop following decreased intestinal calcium absorption [38] and increased urinary calcium excretion [39], leading to a state of relative hypocalcemia. If this statement sounds biologically plausible, however, intact parathyroid hormone (iPTH) levels have not been found to be elevated with the modern assays, even in patients treated with high GC doses [40]. It may be that the hyperparathyroidism state is linked to a stronger sensitivity of bone cells to PTH [41,42] or to an adulteration of the calcium-sensing receptor of parathyroid cells by GCs. GCs might also stimulate osteoclastic bone resorption by concurrently increasing the production of the receptor activator of nuclear factor kappaB ligand (RANKL) by human osteoblastic lineage cells [43] and by rapidly and markedly decreasing the circulating levels of its decoy receptor osteoprotegerin (OPG) [43–45]. RANKL binds to its receptor RANK, which is

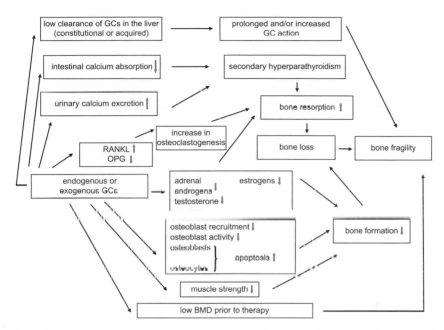

Fig. 4. Several factors acting alone or synergistically in the development of glucocorticoid-induced osteoporosis. OPG, osteoprotegerin; RANKL, receptor activator of NF-κB ligand.

expressed on osteoclast precursors and mature osteoclasts, promoting osteo-clastogenesis. The binding of OPG to RANKL avoids the binding of RANKL to RANK and so inhibits osteoclastogenesis. The marked decrease in OPG circulating levels that is provoked by GC administration as soon as the first 2 weeks, linked to the increased production of RANKL, will lead to rapid stimulation of osteoclastogenesis with early enhanced osteoclastic activity [43–45]. This process could explain the fast bone loss that occurs soon after initiation of GC therapy. Further studies dealing with the OPG/RANKL/RANK system are urgently needed for better understanding of the mechanisms of bone resorption in GC-OP as compared with post-menopausal OP.

GCs also have a direct detrimental action on osteoblasts [37 46] possibly through an impairment of their recruitment and activity, as well as an in-crease in osteoblasts' and osteocytes' apoptosis [47]. Cancellous bone forma-tion, but also cortical bone formation, is impaired, which could explain the increased fracture risk not only at the spine but also at the hip [48]. The ef-fects of GCs on osteocytes may not be restricted to provoking cell death; perhaps, and more importantly, they could lead viable cells to modify their microenvironment. The size of osteocyte lacunae has been found to be in-creased, and a sphere of hypomineralized bone is generated surrounding the lacunae [49]. This observation is reminiscent of the histologic description of P. Meunier and colleagues [50] many years ago in hyperparathyroidism.

Such a periosteocytic resorption could result in local changes in bone resistance.

Hormonal changes

In postmenopausal women, the depression of the hypothalamic-pituitary-gonadal axis provoked by GCs induces decreased serum levels of estradiol, androstenedione, dehydroepiandrosterone sulfate, and progesterone [51]. The role of these hormones in BMD maintenance and bone mechanical resistance is well recognized [52,53]. Testosterone levels have been reported to be low in males chronically treated with GCs [54]. However, estradiol levels have also consistently been found to be low in GC-treated men [55]. It is currently well accepted that, even in males, estradiol rather than testosterone is the more active hormone in maintaining a positive bone balance [56].

Moreover, high GC doses, but not low doses, can provoke sarcopenia, which could cause some bone loss [57].

Bone histomorphometry

Histomorphometrically, low-dose GCs induced a marked decrease in trabecular bone volume and a thinning of the trabeculae as compared with sex- and age-matched controls [37,58–62]. A profound depression of the mineral apposition rate has been observed after tetracycline double labeling [37]. The surfaces of trabecular resorption were much less increased, in frank contrast with postmenopausal OP, in which increased resorption rapidly led to a decline in trabecular number with perforations of the plates [62]. However, with higher GC doses, a loss of trabeculae was also observed. This finding is consistent with an increased bone turnover and resorption [33,61,62]. As already mentioned, trabecular changes might also involve osteocytes' environment. Recent experimental work in mice has shown an increase in the size of the osteocyte lacunae, with reduced mineral-to-matrix ratio determined by Raman microspectroscopy, which may influence bone mechanical resistance [49,63]. Moreover, an increased cortical porosity has also been observed in long-term (at least 1 year) GC-treated patients [64]. It was primarily due to an increase in the number of Haversian canals rather than to an increase in their size. Given that there was no evidence of increased bone resorption at the time the biopsy was performed, this observation would be consistent with a transitory increase in activation frequency soon after initiation of GC therapy, along with a longer-term reduction in bone formation at the level of the bone multicellular unit. The net result is a failure to fill in the formerly resorbed cavities [64]. A significant disruption of trabecular bone microarchitecture, an increase in cortical porosity, and (presumably) an increased size of osteocyte lacunae, all occurring in a short period in patients who are treated with high doses of GC, could explain a rapid increase in bone fragility. The thinning of the trabeculae that remain interconnected, along with the maintenance of bone microarchitecture in

GC-OP (at least after low GC doses), may be central to the rapid resurgence of osteoblastic activity, resulting in a positive bone tissue balance. These factors may also be central to the renewed increase in BMD and to the rapid decrease in fracture risk observed after curative surgical intervention of Cushing's syndrome or after weaning from GC therapy [4,37,65,66].

General measures for management of glucocorticoid-induced osteoporosis

All men and premenopausal and postmenopausal women suffering from a condition that necessitates the prescription of GCs at a dose greater than 5 to 7.5 mg equivalent prednisone per day for at least 3 months should undergo a medical work-up for detection of risk factors for OP. The check-up should include an appraisal in the past history of factors potentially accompanied by low BMD, such as retarded puberty (an incorrigible factor), low calcium intake in the diet, sedentary lifestyle (usually linked to the severity of the condition justifying GC therapy), and smoking and alcohol habits, which are frequently increased in chronic debilitating diseases (all potentially corrigible factors). Laboratory testing should include measurements of fasting serum calcium, phosphate, creatinine, alkaline phosphatase, total protein, and urinary calcium over creatinine. Testing should also ideally include 25-hydroxyvitamin D3 (25OHD) and a parameter of bone resorption such as serum C-telopeptide. BMD of the spine and the hip should be measured by dual energy x-ray absorptiometry.

In GC-OP, there is some evidence that fractures may happen at a BMD level higher than the conventional value of 2.5 standard deviations (T-scores) applied in postmenopausal OP. Hence some have suggested choosing a T-score of -1 to -1.5 as the intervention threshold for therapy in GC-treated patients [67–69].

In GC-treated patients who have chronic diseases, supplemental calcium and vitamin D should be given at a daily dose averaging 800 to 1000 IU/d, particularly in patients avoiding sun exposure (eg, lupus erythematosus disseminated patients) to maintain 25OHD levels above 30 ng/mL and prevent secondary increase of PTH [70]. An increase in physical activity should be recommended, as long as the general health of the patient allows it. In patients after organ transplantation, for example, the author found a positive correlation between total hip bone mineral content (BMC) and Baecke's sport index (Fig. 5) [71]. Moreover, a trend toward lower values of fat content and fat percentage at trunk level was observed in transplanted patients with high activity [71]. It is well known that truncal obesity constitutes a risk factor for cardiovascular diseases [72].

Therapy

Beyond the general measures advocated in the preceding section, it is advisable to use the lowest GC doses or even to withdraw GC therapy as early

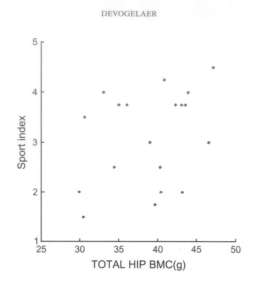

Fig. 5. Correlation between Baecke's sport index and total hip BMC in 19 patients posttransplantation ($R = .48$; $P < .05$). (*From* Cordier P, Decruynaere C, Devogelaer JP. Bone mineral density in posttransplantation patients: effects of physical activity. Transplant Proc 2000;32:411–4; with permission.)

as possible, to prevent structural damage to the skeleton [61,62] and hence to expect some protection of the BMD and even a trend toward recovery [37,65,66]. However, no truly safe dose exists, and weaning the patient from GCs is rarely possible. The choice of the lowest GC dose possible is common sense and depends on the individual practitioner's decision. Grossly, there is no real evidence-based indication of a precise dose of GC in the numerous conditions necessitating this therapy, even though many recommendations for the prevention of GC-OP now exist [73–76]. Alternate-day therapy helps to maintain growth in children. However, BMD is not preserved [77,78]; the continuing bone loss is probably caused by the persistent depression of the secretion of adrenal androgens on the day off GCs [79]. The role of the adrenal androgens in the maintenance of BMD has already been underlined [52]. Inhaled GCs are increasingly used in therapy for chronic obstructive pulmonary diseases. Whether their use is devoid of adverse skeletal effects is still debated [17,80]. Intravenous pulse dosing of methylprednisolone (as much as 1 g) does not appear to be deleterious for BMD [18]. However, this would not be the case if the doses were repeated too frequently.

Deflazacort was reputed to be less detrimental to bone than equipotent doses of prednisone [13–15]. Moreover, in children, it was less deleterious to growth [81,82]. Its peculiar behavior was attributed to several mechanisms [83]. However, some controversy still exists about its real equipotency to prednisone [16,84].

A rapid weaning from GCs may rarely be considered; moreover, even when bone is less threatened by low daily doses (equal to or less than 5 to

7.5 mg equivalent prednisolone per day), there is no definitely safe dose as far as bone integrity is concerned. Therefore, considerable room still exists for pharmacologic preventive therapy in GC-OP. Several compounds aimed at protecting bone have been studied in randomized trials. They include antiresorptive agents such as calcium, vitamin D, and its more polar metabolites, hormonal therapy, calcitonin, bisphosphonate, and promotors of bone formation, such as fluoride salts and parathyroid hormone

Antiresorptive agents

Calcium and vitamin D
No data in the literature suggests that calcium supplementation alone can prevent the rapid bone loss observed in patients who are starting GC therapy [85]. Not a single study addressed the use of calcium alone in fracture prevention of GC-OP.

Plain cholecalciferol (400 IU/d to 100,000 IU/wk) [86–91], dihydrotachystcrol (0.1 mg every other day) [92], calcidiol (35 to 40 µg/d) [93–96], calcitriol (0.5 to 1.0 µg/d) [97–100], and alfacalcidol (0.5 to 1.0 µg/d) [101–103] plus calcium were able to impair bone loss, and they proved to have a superior effect on BMD compared with calcium alone [104,105]. Only one small study (controlled but not double blind; total number of patients N = 85) compared the effects of plain vitamin D on BMD with those of a more polar derivative [103]. Alfacalcidol (1.0 µg + 500 mg calcium per day) could produce a larger increase in lumbar BMD than plain cholecalciferol (1000 IU + 500 mg calcium per day), but the differential effect on vertebral fractures remained conjectural. No difference was observed on hip BMD or on fracture rate [103]. It should be remembered that the risk for hypercalciuria or hypercalcemia is larger with more polar vitamin D metabolites than with cholecalciferol. It might be suggested, therefore, that calcium supplementation plus plain vitamin D3 is a therapeutic modality in association with more potent molecules (eg, bisphosphonates), and that their isolated use should be reserved for patients who are on GC doses lower than 7.5 mg equivalent prednisolone per day, or during the first 3 months of therapy, if treatment with GCs is short lived [76].

Hormone replacement therapy
Because hypogonadism frequently occurs on high-dose GC therapy, hormone replacement therapy (HRT) could be considered in postmenopausal women and in men, provided no contraindication to its use exists. If HRT has been shown to be capable of preventing BMD loss, there is no trial that has assessed fracture prevention in women or in men [57,106,107]. So far no study exists on tibolone in the prevention of GC-OP. It is unlikely, however, that HRT or tibolone could be recommended over the long term, following the Women's Health Initiative study and the premature cessation of the long-term intervention on fractures with tibolone study for

safety reasons [108,109]. If testosterone-replacement therapy in men was able to counteract bone loss and myopathy, nandrolone decanoate had a positive effect only on muscle wasting [57]. HRT in men should only be envisaged in the case of low androgen levels. No study exists so far of raloxifene in post-menopausal women on GCs. In women who are suffering from breast cancer and otherwise treated by GCs, tamoxifen could be protective for BMD [110]. A study has also shown a positive effect of medroxyprogesterone acetate on bone loss [111].

Prasterone, the synthetic form of dehydroepiandrosterone, at a dose of 200 mg per day, not only prevented bone loss but also significantly increased lumbar and total hip BMD in a small group of female lupus patients who were receiving GC therapy (≤ 10 mg/day equivalent prednisone) [112]. Further studies on HRT are urgently needed.

Calcitonin

Calcitonin administered as parenteral subcutaneous injections or intranasal spray has been shown to be capable of preventing bone loss in patients treated with GCs, at least at the spine and the distal radius, but not at the femoral neck [113]. This was the conclusion of a recent Cochrane review of nine trials including 221 patients randomized to calcitonin and 220 to placebo [98,113–121]. The populations involved suffered from rheumatic conditions such as polymyalgia rheumatica, temporal arteritis or rheumatoid arthritis [98,119–121], chronic obstructive pulmonary disease [114, 115], and asthma [116,117]. Injectable calcitonin was administered in three trials [114,116,119]. The Cochrane reviewers classified four trials as prevention trials and five as treatment trials, based on the duration of GC therapy (<3 or >3 months) before starting calcitonin [113]. Curiously, no dose-response effect occurred with calcitonin. But the greatest difference in BMD between treated and control groups was observed in the trial that used subcutaneous injections [116], consistent with a greater bioavailability of the injectable form of calcitonin. Moreover, its beneficial effect may be greater in patients who have taken GCs for longer than 3 months. No demonstrated effectiveness of calcitonin in the prevention of fractures associated with GC-OP was found; however, the sample size of the trials was not adequate to assess fracture rate, even by pooling several trials [113]. Calcitonin could be considered as an alternative treatment for GC-OP, particularly in patients who have been taking GCs for longer than 3 months [113]. Theoretic advantages of calcitonin are not requiring oral administration, which could add to the digestive loading of oral medicines already taken by rheumatic patients, and probably having analgesic properties [83].

Bisphosphonates
Etidronate disodium. Cyclical intermittent etidronate (400 mg/d for 14 days, followed by calcium 500 mg/d every 3 months) was able significantly to increase lumbar BMD in both prevention and treatment studies. The effect on

the hip BMD was less marked [87,122–130]. A minority of studies have reported on fracture rate [87,124,125,129]. In only one study, a significant reduction in the proportion of postmenopausal women with new vertebral fractures was observed in the etidronate group versus placebo, whereas the fracture rate increased in men [125]. In another study, more symptomatic fractures were observed in the treated group [124]. However, it should be noted that all these trials were inadequately sized to assess antifracture efficacy.

Clodronate. Oral clodronate (1600 mg/d and 2400 mg/d) significantly increased lumbar BMD after 1 year in patients who had already been taking GCs for at least 6 months (mean duration more than 6.5 years). At the hip, only the dose of 2400 mg significantly increased BMD [131]. No data were available as far as fracture rate was concerned. Tolerance was similar to that of placebo [131]. Intramuscular clodronate (100 mg, once weekly) was able to maintain BMD at the lumbar spine, at the hip, and in the total body for 4 years. By contrast, a large loss (−6.54% to −8.06%) was seen in the control group in patients suffering from rheumatoid or psoriatic arthritis who had started prednisone within the previous 100 days [132]. A decrease of 37% in the vertebral fracture risk was observed in the actively treated group. Eight percent of patients dropped out because of local pain at the site of injection [132].

Pamidronate disodium. For primary prevention, pamidronate was administered intravenously to patients starting long-term GC therapy at a dose of at least 10 mg/d of prednisolone. An initial 90-mg dose of pamidronate, whether given singly or followed at 3-month intervals by 30-mg doses for 1 year, produced similar increases in lumbar BMD and hip BMD, versus a significant loss in the control group [133].

Oral pamidronate at a dose of 100 mg/d (plus calcium and vitamin D) was able to prevent bone loss at the spine in premenopausal women who were put on high-dose GCs, as compared with calcium–vitamin D alone [134].

Alendronate sodium. Alendronate was administered orally at a dose of 2.5 mg, 5 mg, or 10 mg, plus 800 to 1000 mg of elemental calcium and 250 to 500 IU of vitamin D daily, versus placebo (plus the same supplementations) to patients who had been put on GCs less than 4 months ago, 4 to 12 months ago, or longer ago than 12 months [135]. A significant increase in lumbar BMD was observed from baseline in the 5-mg and 10-mg alendronate groups (+2.1% and +2.9%, respectively), but the gain was not significant in the 2.5-mg group. An insignificant loss occurred in the placebo group. A more marked (albeit still not significant) bone loss was observed in the group of patients who had been taking GCs for the shorter period. Femoral neck BMD increased significantly in the two higher alendronate dosage groups, versus a significant loss in the placebo group. No significant effect on the vertebral and nonvertebral fracture rates was observed in the two higher alendronate dosage groups versus the placebo group [135]. Continuation of the study for 1 more year showed a continued increase in BMD. Fewer patients who were taking alendronate versus placebo developed new morphometric vertebral fractures after 2 years (0.7% versus 6.8%; $P < .05$). No fracture occurred in men in either group [31]. Both alendronate (10 mg/d) and calcitriol (0.5 μg/d) were able to protect bone at the lumbar spine (-0.7% and -1.0%, respectively) and at the hip (-1.7% and -2.1%, respectively) versus a loss of respectively -3.2% and -6.2% in the control group in the first year after cardiac transplantation [136]. No significant difference in the vertebral fracture rate was observed. Hypercalciuria was evident in 27% of the patients in the calcitriol group versus 7% in the alendronate group ($P < .01$) [137]. The observed necessity of monitoring calciuria does not favor using calcitriol for this indication.

Risedronate sodium. The results of two studies on risedronate in GC-OP, one a primary prevention study of patients who had been taking GCs for 3 months or less [138] and one a treatment study of patients who had been taking GCs for more than 6 months [29], were pooled in a third paper to increase the statistical power to assess antifracture efficacy [30]. Risedronate at a dose of 2.5 mg/d or 5 mg/d was administered versus placebo for 1 year in 518 ambulatory men and women, 18 to 85 years of age, who were receiving 7.5 mg prednisone daily or greater. In the overall population, there was a small but significant increase in both lumbar BMD ($+1.9$%; $P < .001$ versus baseline and placebo) and BMD at the femoral neck ($+1.3$%; $P < .01$ versus baseline and $P < .001$ versus placebo). On a dose of 2.5 mg, the increase was only significant at the lumbar spine. A significant reduction in the incidence of morphometric vertebral fractures was observed in patients who were taking 5 mg (-70%) and 2.5 mg (-58%) risedronate, as compared with placebo ($P = .01$ and .08, respectively). In individual studies [29,138], only a trend toward a reduction in vertebral fracture rate was observed. This positive effect of 5 mg risedronate was evidenced across the various conditions necessitating GC therapy, as well as in both patients with and without prevalent vertebral fracture. Fewer patients in the risedronate groups experienced multiple vertebral fractures than in the placebo group. No significant effect was observed on nonvertebral fractures. Interestingly, the subgroup of men underwent a significant decrease (-82.4%; $P = .008$) in the incidence of vertebral fractures in the pooled risedronate groups [32].

A study restricted to patients suffering from a single condition (ie, rheumatoid arthritis) and treated with at least 2.5 mg prednisolone per day has followed BMD on risedronate (2.5 mg/d or cyclical 15 mg/d for 15 days, followed by placebo daily for 10 weeks) and on placebo. During the third year, no active drug was provided [136]. Two years of risedronate maintained BMD at the spine and at the hip, whereas the placebo group had significant bone loss. Risedronate discontinuation resulted in bone loss at all skeletal sites (Fig. 6). This observation supports the need for continuous treatment

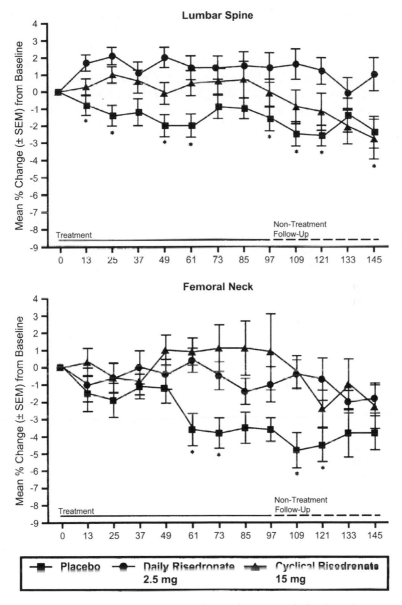

Fig. 6. Mean (± standard error of the mean) changes in BMD at the lumbar spine (*top panel*) and at the femoral neck (*bottom panel*) from baseline to week 145 in the study of daily 2.5-mg risedronate, cyclical 15-mg risedronate, administered for 97 weeks versus placebo, followed by 1 year without therapy. (*From* Eastell R, Devogelaer JP, Peel NFA, et al. Prevention of bone loss with risedronate in glucocorticoid-treated rheumatoid arthritis patients. Osteoporos Int 2000;11:331–7; with permission.)

with risedronate to prevent bone loss for as long as GC therapy must be maintained [138].

More recently, studies pertaining to the role of zoledronic acid in GC-OP have been initiated. This drug has the dual advantage of the intravenous route of administration (which is convenient in patients who are already taking several drugs, such as those suffering from rheumatic conditions) and of annual administration [139].

No data exist yet on ibandronate or denosumab in GC-OP.

Promoters of bone formation

In GC-OP, bone formation is impaired, and a thinning of trabeculae has been observed histomorphometrically [37,46,47,58–62].

Common sense appears to dictate prescribing promoters of bone formation to prevent the adverse consequences of GC therapy for bone.

In numerous studies involving GC-OP, fluoride salts therapy has demonstrated an equivalent efficacy in increasing lumbar BMD to its efficacy in postmenopausal OP [86,140–146]. These studies have not assessed the antifracture efficacy of fluoride in GC-OP, however.

In a small trial of 1 year's duration, human PTH (hPTH) [1–34] was shown dramatically to increase lumbar BMD in 28 postmenopausal women who were on concurrent estrogen replacement therapy and a stable dose of prednisone (mean dosage 5–20 mg/d) for at least 1 year (+11.8%), as compared with 23 women receiving estrogen therapy only [147]. A leveling off of lumbar BMD occurred in the second year. At the hip, the increase in BMD was more modest (+2% from the start) after 1 year, but the hip BMD still increased in the second year after discontinuation of hPTH (+4.7%) [147,148]. Serum levels of RANKL increased rapidly within 1 month of hPTH therapy, peaked at more than 250% above baseline values at 3 months, and remained elevated (>150% above initial values) for the rest of the year of therapy. OPG levels decreased from 6 months (−23%), and the nadir was attained at 12 months (−45%). After discontinuation of hPTH, both values returned to baseline [149]. These data support the notion that daily administered hPTH [1–34] rapidly stimulates osteoblast function. The delayed and reduced suppression of OPG could lead to some osteoclast activation and rebalancing of bone remodeling [149]. Large studies of the action of teriparatide (hPTH 1-34) in the prevention and therapy of GC-OP are currently in progress.

So far no study of strontium ranelate and GCs exists.

As in postmenopausal OP, there is currently no rationale for either a therapeutic regimen combining two antiresorptive agents (with the remarkable exception of calcium and vitamin D) or a simultaneous association of antiresorptive-anabolic agents. No proof exists that the increased costs entailed by their concomitant administration will lead to an increase in therapeutic efficacy, as far as fracture prevention is concerned. Studies are therefore still needed to determine, as for postmenopausal OP, which combined therapy regimen (if any) could be proposed, following which alternation of the two agents, and for which particular indication.

No data exist in the literature regarding the duration of therapy for GC-OP. Given the mechanisms of development of GC-OP (see Fig. 6) and the rapid waning of the therapeutic efficacy of most drugs, it appears logical to maintain preventive therapy, whatever the chosen preventive means, as long as GCs are prescribed at a dose of at least 7.5 mg equivalent prednisolone daily. There should be no indication to prolong therapy unduly after discontinuing GCs, because more than circumstantial evidence points to at least partial spontaneous recovery of the skeleton after cessation of GC excess [37,65,66]. An exception may be patients who have BMD levels below the osteoporotic threshold (ie, ≤ -2.5 T-scores).

New alternatives to the currently existent GCs, preserving their anti-inflammatory properties with fewer side effects, could be developed in the future [150]. In the meantime, new therapeutic agents that permit the use of lower doses of concomitant GCs or whose use is accompanied by smaller degrees of bone loss, such as anti–tumor necrosis factor α agents in rheumatoid arthritis [151] or possibly tacrolimus in organ transplantation [152], should be tested for their antiosteoporotic adjuvant action.

Summary

GCs constitute a therapeutic class largely used in clinical medicine for the curative or supportive treatment of various conditions involving the intervention of numerous medical specialties. Beyond their favorable therapeutic effects, GCs almost invariably provoke bone loss and a rapid increase in bone fragility, with its host of fractures. Men and postmenopausal women constitute a preferential target for the bone complications of GCs. The premenopausal status is not, however, a shelter; bone loss also happens in young women who are on GCs. Exposure to GCs yields a fracture risk exceeding the risk conferred by a low BMD per se. Therefore, some reason exists to settle the BMD threshold for therapeutic intervention not at -2.5 T-scores but at -1.0 or -1.5 T-scores, even if no prospective randomized trial so far endorses that opinion. Nowadays, bisphosphonate therapy should be proposed to every patient at risk for fragility fracture, along with calcium and vitamin D supplementation. Studies of other therapeutic modalities (eg, promoters of bone formation) are in progress.

Acknowledgments

The author is grateful to Marie-Christine Hallot for her helpful assistance in typing the manuscript.

References

[1] Hench PS, Kendall EC, Slocumb CH, et al. The effect of a hormone of the adrenal cortex (17-hydroxy-11-dehydrocorticosterone: compound E) and of pituitary adrenocorticotropic hormone on rheumatoid arthritis. Preliminary report. Proc Staff Meet Mayo Clin 1949; 24(8):181–97.

[2] Howell DS, Ragan C. The course of rheumatoid arthritis during four years of induced hyperadrenalism (IHA). Medicine (Baltimore) 1956;35(2):83–119.

[3] Kanis JA, Johansson H, Oden A, et al. A meta-analysis of prior corticosteroid use and fracture risk. J Bone Miner Res 2004;19(6):893–9.

[4] van Staa TP, Leufkens HGM, Abenhaim L, et al. Use of oral corticosteroids and risk of fractures. J Bone Miner Res 2000;15(6):993–1000.

[5] Curtis JR, Westfall AO, Allison JJ, et al. Longitudinal patterns in the prevention of osteoporosis in glucocorticoid-treated patients. Arthritis Rheum 2005;52(8):2485–94.

[6] van Staa TP, Cooper C, Leufkens HGM, et al. Children and the risk of fractures caused by oral corticosteroids. J Bone Miner Res 2003;18(5):913–8.

[7] Hahn TJ, Boisseau VC, Avioli LV. Effect of chronic corticosteroid administration on diaphyseal and metaphyseal bone mass. J Clin Endocrinol Metab 1974;39(2):274–82.

[8] Nagant de Deuxchaisnes C, Devogelaer JP, Esselinckx W, et al. The effect of low dosage glucocorticoids on bone mass in rheumatoid arthritis: a cross-sectional and a longitudinal study using single photon absorptiometry. Adv Exp Med Biol 1984;171:209–39.

[9] Maldague B, Malghem J, Nagant de Deuxchaisnes C. Radiological aspects of glucocorticoid-induced bone disease. Adv Exp Med Biol 1984;171:155–90.

[10] Reid IR, Evans MC, Wattie DJ, et al. Bone mineral density of the proximal femur and lumbar spine in glucocorticoid-treated asthmatic patients. Osteoporos Int 1992;2(2):103–5.

[11] Albright F. Cushing's syndrome. Harvey Lect 1942;38:123–86.

[12] Cooper MS, Rabbitt EH, Goddard PE, et al. Osteoblastic 11 β-hydroxysteroid dehydrogenase type 1 activity increases with age and glucocorticoid exposure. J Bone Miner Res 2002; 17(6):979–86.

[13] Devogelaer JP, Huaux JP, Dufour JP, et al. Bone-sparing action of deflazacort versus equipotent doses of prednisone: a double-blind study in males with rheumatoid arthritis. In: Christiansen C, Johansen JS, Riis BJ, editors. Osteoporosis 1987. Viborg, Denmark: Norhaven A/S; 1987. p. 1014–5.

[14] Olgaard K, Storm T, van Wowern N, et al. Glucocorticoid-induced osteoporosis in the lumbar spine, forearm, and mandible of nephrotic patients: a double-blind study on the high-dose, long-term effects of prednisone versus deflazacort. Calcif Tissue Int 1992;50(6):490–7.

[15] Gray RES, Doherty SM, Galloway J, et al. A double-blind study of deflazacort and prednisone in patients with chronic inflammatory disorders. Arthritis Rheum 1991;34(3): 287–95.

[16] Cacoub P, Chemlal K, Khalifa P, et al. Deflazacort versus prednisone in patients with giant cell arteritis: effects on bone mass loss. J Rheumatol 2001;28(11):2474–9.

[17] Richy F, Bousquet J, Ehrlich GE, et al. Inhaled corticosteroids effects on bone in asthmatic and COPD patients: a quantitative systematic review. Osteoporos Int 2003;14(3):179–90.

[18] Frediani B, Falsetti P, Bisogno S, et al. Effects of high dose methylprednisolone pulse therapy on bone mass and biochemical markers of bone metabolism in patients with active rheumatoid arthritis: a 12-month randomized prospective controlled study. J Rheumatol 2004;31(6):1083–7.

[19] Dovio A, Perazzolo L, Osella G, et al. Immediate fall of bone formation and transient increase in bone resorption in the course of high-dose, short-term glucocorticoid therapy in young patients with multiple sclerosis. J Clin Endocrinol Metab 2004;89(10):4923–8.

[20] van Staa TP, Leufkens HGM, Abenhaim L, et al. Oral corticosteroids and fracture risk: relationship to daily and cumulative doses. Rheumatology 2000;39(12):1383–9.

[21] van Staa TP, Laan RF, Barton IP, et al. Bone density threshold and other predictors of vertebral fracture in patients receiving oral glucocorticoid therapy. Arthritis Rheum 2003; 48(11):3224–9.

[22] Reid DM, Kennedy NSJ, Smith MA, et al. Total body calcium in rheumatoid arthritis: effects of disease activity and corticosteroid treatment. BMJ 1982;285(6338):330–2.

[23] Wolthers OD, Pedersen S. Short term linear growth in asthmatic children during treatment with prednisolone. BMJ 1990;301(6744):145–8.

[24] Leonard MB, Zemel BS. Pediatric gastroenterology and nutrition. Current concepts in pediatric bone disease. Pediatr Clin North Am 2002;49(1):143–73.

[25] Boot AM, de Jongste JC, Verberne AAPH, et al. Bone mineral density and bone metabolism of prepubertal children with asthma after long-term treatment with inhaled corticosteroids. Pediatr Pulmonol 1997;24(6):379–84.

[26] Hochberg Z. Mechanisms of steroid impairment of growth. Horm Res 2002;58(Suppl 1): 33–8.

[27] Saville PD, Kharmosh O. Osteoporosis of rheumatoid arthritis: influence of age, sex and corticosteroids. Arthritis Rheum 1967;10(5):423–30.

[28] Jardinet D, Lefèbvre C, Depresseux G, et al. Longitudinal analysis of bone mineral density in pre-menopausal female systemic lupus erythematosus patients: deleterious role of glucocorticoid therapy at the lumbar spine. Rheumatology 2000;39(4):389–92.

[29] Reid DM, Hughes RA, Laan RFJM, et al. Efficacy and safety of daily risedronate in the treatment of corticosteroid-induced osteoporosis in men and women: a randomized trial. J Bone Miner Res 2000;15(6):1006–13.

[30] Wallach S, Cohen S, Reid DM, et al. Effects of risedronate treatment on bone density and vertebral fracture in patients on corticosteroid therapy. Calcif Tissue Int 2000; 67(4):277–85.

[31] Adachi JD, Saag KG, Delmas PD, et al. Two-year effects of alendronate on bone mineral density and vertebral fracture in patients receiving glucocorticoids. A randomized, double-blind, placebo-controlled extension trial. Arthritis Rheum 2001;44(1):202–11.

[32] Reid DM, Adami S, Devogelaer J-P, et al. Risedronate increases bone density and reduces vertebral fracture risk within one year in men on corticosteroid therapy. Calcif Tissue Int 2001;69(4):242–7.

[33] Prummel MF, Wiersinga WM, Lips P, et al. The course of biochemical parameters of bone turnover during treatment with corticosteroids. J Clin Endocrinol Metab 1991; 72(2):382–6.

[34] Kozower M, Veatch L, Kaplan MM. Decreased clearance of prednisolone, a factor in the development of corticosteroid side effects. J Clin Endocrinol Metab 1974;38(3): 407–12.

[35] Stevens A, Ray DW, Zeggini E, et al. Glucocorticoid sensitivity is determined by a specific glucocorticoid receptor haplotype. J Clin Endocrinol Metab 2004;89(2):892–7.

[36] Fucik RF, Kukreja SC, Hargis GK, et al. Effect of glucocorticoids on function of the parathyroid glands in man. J Clin Endocrinol Metab 1975;40(1):152–5.

[37] Bressot C, Meunier PJ, Chapuy MC, et al. Histomorphometric profile, pathophysiology and reversibility of corticosteroid-induced osteoporosis. Metab Bone Dis Relat Res 1979; 1:303–11.

[38] Morris HA, Need AG, O'Loughlin PD, et al. Malabsorption of calcium in corticosteroid-induced osteoporosis. Calcif Tissue Int 1990;46(5):305–8.

[39] Suzuki Y, Ichikawa Y, Saito E, et al. Importance of increased urinary calcium excretion in the development of secondary hyperparathyroidism of patients under glucocorticoid therapy. Metabolism 1983;32(2):151–6.

[40] Paz-Pacheco E, El-Hajj Fuleihan G, Leboff MS. Intact parathyroid hormone levels are not elevated in glucocorticoid-treated subjects. J Bone Miner Res 1995;10(11):1713–8.

[41] Silve C, Fritsch J, Grosse B, et al. Corticosteroid-induced changes in the responsiveness of human osteoblast-like cells to parathyroid hormone. Bone Miner 1989;6(1):65–75.

[42] Rodan SB, Fischer MK, Egan JJ, et al. The effect of dexamethasone on parathyroid hormone stimulation of adenylate cyclase in ROS 17/2.8 cells. Endocrinology 1984;115(3): 951–8.

[43] Hofbauer LC, Gori F, Riggs BL, et al. Stimulation of osteoprotegerin ligand and inhibition of osteoprotegerin production by glucocorticoids in human osteoblastic lineage cells: potential paracrine mechanisms of glucocorticoid-induced osteoporosis. Endocrinology 1999;140(10):4382–9.

[44] Sasaki N, Kusano E, Ando Y, et al. Glucocorticoid decreases circulating osteoprotegerin (OPG): possible mechanism for glucocorticoid induced osteoporosis. Nephrol Dial Transplant 2001;16(3):479–82.

[45] von Tirpitz C, Epp S, Klaus J, et al. Effect of systemic glucocorticoid therapy on bone metabolism and the osteoprotegerin system in patients with active Crohn's disease. Eur J Gastroenterol Hepatol 2003;15(11):1165–70.

[46] Godschalk MF, Downs RW. Effect of short-term glucocorticoids on serum osteocalcin in healthy young men. J Bone Miner Res 1988;3(1):113–5.

[47] Weinstein RS, Jilka RL, Parfitt AM, et al. Inhibition of osteoblastogenesis and promotion of apoptosis of osteoblasts and osteocytes by glucocorticoids. Potential mechanisms of their deleterious effects on bone. J Clin Invest 1998;102(2):274–82.

[48] Schorlemmer S, Ignatius A, Claes L, et al. Inhibition of cortical and cancellous bone formation in glucocorticoid-treated OVX sheep. Bone 2005;37(4):491–6.

[49] Lane NE. New observations on bone fragility with glucocorticoid treatment. Results from an in vivo animal model. J Musculoskelet Neuronal Interact 2005;5(4):331–2.

[50] Meunier P, Bernard J, Vignon G. La mesure de l'élargissement périostéocytaire appliquée au diagnostic des hyperparathyroïdies. Path Biol (Paris) 1971;19(7–8):371–8.

[51] Montecucco C, Caporali R, Caprotti P, et al. Sex hormones and bone metabolism in postmenopausal rheumatoid arthritis treated with two different glucocorticoids. J Rheumatol 1992;19(12):1895–900.

[52] Devogelaer JP, Crabbé J, Nagant de Deuxchaisnes C. Bone mineral density in Addison's disease: evidence for an effect of adrenal androgens on bone mass. BMJ 1987;294(6575): 798–800.

[53] Cauley JA, Robbins J, Chen Z, et al. Effects of estrogen plus progestin on risk of fracture and bone mineral density: the Women's Health Initiative randomized trial. JAMA 2003; 290(13):1729–38.

[54] MacAdams MR, White RH, Chipps BE. Reduction of serum testosterone levels during chronic glucocorticoid therapy. Ann Intern Med 1986;104(5):648–51.

[55] Hampson G, Bhargava N, Cheung J, et al. Low circulating estradiol and adrenal androgens concentrations in men on glucocorticoids: a potential contributory factor in steroid-induced osteoporosis. Metabolism 2002;51(11):1458–62.

[56] Riggs BL, Khosla S, Melton LJ 3rd. A unitary model for involutional osteoporosis: estrogen deficiency causes both type I and type II osteoporosis in postmenopausal women and contributes to bone loss in aging men. J Bone Miner Res 1998;13(5):763–73.

[57] Crawford BAL, Liu PY, Kean MT, et al. Randomized placebo-controlled trial of androgen effects on muscle and bone in men requiring long-term systemic glucocorticoid treatment. J Clin Endocrinol Metab 2003;88(7):3167–76.

[58] Dempster DW. Perspectives. Bone histomorphometry in glucocorticoid-induced osteoporosis. J Bone Miner Res 1989;4(2):137–41.

[59] Stellon AJ, Webb A, Compston JE. Bone histomorphometry and structure in corticosteroid treated chronic active hepatitis. Gut 1988;29:378–84.

[60] Aaron JE, Francis RM, Peacock M, et al. Contrasting microanatomy of idiopathic and corticosteroid-induced osteoporosis. Clin Orthop 1989;243:294–305.

[61] Chappard D, Legrand E, Basle MF, et al. Altered trabecular architecture induced by corticosteroids: a bone histomorphometric study. J Bone Miner Res 1996;11(5): 676–85.

[62] Dalle Carbonare L, Arlot ME, Chavassieux PM, et al. Comparison of trabecular bone microarchitecture and remodeling in glucocorticoid-induced and postmenopausal osteoporosis. J Bone Miner Res 2001;16(1):97–103.

[63] Lane NE, Yao W, Balooch M, et al. Glucocorticoid-treated mice have localized changes in trabecular bone material properties and osteocyte lacunar size that are not observed in placebo-treated or estrogen-deficient mice. J Bone Miner Res 2006; 21(3):466–76.

[64] Vedi S, Elkin SL, Compston JE. A histomorphometric study of cortical bone of the iliac crest in patients treated with glucocorticoids. Calcif Tissue Int 2005;77:79–83.

[65] Pocock NA, Eisman JA, Dunstan CR, et al. Recovery from steroid-induced osteoporosis. Ann Intern Med 1987;107:319–23.

[66] Laan RFJM, van Riel PLCM, van de Putte LBA, et al. Low-dose prednisolone induces rapid reversible axial bone loss in patients with rheumatoid arthritis. Ann Intern Med 1993;119:963–8.

[67] Abadie EC, Devogelaer J-P, Ringe JD, et al. Recommendations for the registration of agents to be used in the prevention and treatment of glucocorticoid-induced osteoporosis: updated recommendations from the Group for the Respect of Ethics and Excellence in Science. Semin Arthritis Rheum 2005;35:1–4.

[68] Bone and Tooth Society of Great Britain, Royal College of Physicians, and National Osteoporosis Society. Guidelines on the prevention and treatment of glucocorticoid-induced osteoporosis. London: Royal College of Physicians; 2003.

[69] Sambrook PN. How to prevent steroid induced osteoporosis. Ann Rheum Dis 2005;64: 176 8.

[70] Holick MF. Vitamin D. Clinical Review in Bone and Mineral Metabolism 2002;1(3/4): 181–207.

[71] Cordier P, Decruynaere C, Devogelaer JP. Bone mineral density in postransplantation patients: effects of physical activity. Transplant Proc 2000;32:411–4.

[72] Mahony JF, Savdie E, Caterson RJ, et al. The natural history of cadaveric renal allografts beyond ten years. Transplant Proc 1986;18:135–7.

[73] American College of Rheumatology Task Force on Osteoporosis Guidelines. Recommendations for the prevention and treatment of glucocorticoid-induced osteoporosis. Arthritis Rheum 1996;39(11):1791–801.

[74] Adler RA, Hochberg MC. Suggested guidelines for evaluation and treatment of glucocorticoid-induced osteoporosis for the department of Veterans Affairs. Arch Intern Med 2003; 163(21):2619–24.

[75] Bone and Tooth Society of Great Britain, National Osteoporosis Society and Royal College of Physicians. Glucocorticoid-induced osteoporosis. Guidelines on prevention and treatment. London: Royal College of Physicians; 2002. Available at http://www.rcplondon. ac.uk/pubs/brochure.aspx?e=89. Accessed October 5, 2006.

[76] Devogelaer JP, Goemaere S, Boonen S, et al. Evidence-based guidelines for the prevention and treatment of glucocorticoid-induced osteoporosis: a consensus document of the Belgian Bone Club. Osteoporos Int 2006;17(1):8–19.

[77] Gluck OS, Murphy WA, Hahn TJ, et al. Bone loss in adults receiving alternate day glucocorticoid therapy. A comparison with daily therapy. Arthritis Rheum 1981; 24(7):892–8.

[78] Rüegsegger P, Medici TC, Anliker M. Corticosteroid-induced bone loss. A longitudinal study of alternate day therapy in patients with bronchial asthma using quantitative computed tomography. Eur J Clin Pharmacol 1983;25:615–20.

[79] Avgerinos PC, Cutler GB, Tsokos GC, et al. Dissociation between cortisol and adrenal androgen secretion in patients receiving alternate day prednisone therapy. J Clin Endocrinol Metab 1987;65:24–9.

[80] van Staa TP, Leufkens HGM, Cooper C. Use of inhaled corticosteroids and risk of fractures. J Bone Miner Res 2001;16:581–8.

[81] Loftus J, Allen R, Hesp R, et al. Randomized, double-blind trial of deflazacort versus prednisone in juvenile chronic (or rheumatoid) arthritis: a relatively bone-sparing effect of deflazacort. Pediatrics 1991;88:428–36.

[82] David J, Loftus J, Hesp R, et al. Spinal and somatic growth in patients with juvenile chronic arthritis treated for up to 2 years with deflazacort. Clin Exp Rheumatol 1992;10(6):621–4.

[83] Devogelaer JP, Manicourt DH, Boutsen Y. Glucocorticoid-induced osteoporosis: prevention and treatment. Curr Top Ster Res 2004;4:217–26.

[84] Devogelaer J-P, Gennari C. Deflazacort in giant cell arteritis. J Rheumatol 2002;29(10): 2244.

[85] Sambrook PN. Corticosteroid osteoporosis: practical implications of recent trials. J Bone Miner Res 2000;15(9):1645–9.

[86] Rickers H, Deding A, Christiansen C, et al. Corticosteroid-induced osteopenia and vitamin D metabolism. Effect of vitamin D_2, calcium phosphate and sodium fluoride administration. Clin Endocrinol (Oxf) 1982;16(4):409–15.

[87] Worth H, Stammen D, Keck E. Therapy of steroid-induced bone loss in adult asthmatics with calcium, vitamin D, and a diphosphonate. Am J Respir Crit Care Med 1994;150(2): 394–7.

[88] Vogelsang H, Ferenci P, Resch H, et al. Prevention of bone mineral loss in patients with Crohn's disease by long-term oral vitamin D supplementation. Eur J Gastroenterol Hepatol 1995;7(7):605–14.

[89] Bernstein CN, Seeger LL, Anton PA, et al. A randomized, placebo-controlled trial of calcium supplementation for decreased bone density in corticosteroid-using patients with inflammatory bowel disease: a pilot study. Aliment Pharmacol Ther 1996;10(5): 777–86.

[90] Buckley LM, Leib ES, Cartularo KS, et al. Calcium and vitamin D3 supplementation prevents bone loss in the spine secondary to low-dose corticosteroids in patients with rheumatoid arthritis. A randomized, double-blind, placebo-controlled trial. Ann Intern Med 1996; 125(12):961–8.

[91] Adachi JD, Bensen WG, Bianchi F, et al. Vitamin D and calcium in the prevention of corticosteroid induced osteoporosis: a 3 year followup. J Rheumatol 1996;23(6): 995–1000.

[92] Bijlsma JWJ, Raymakers JA, Mosch C, et al. Effect of oral calcium and vitamin D on glucocorticoid-induced osteopenia. Clin Exp Rheumatol 1988;6(2):113–9.

[93] Di Munno O, Beghe F, Favini P, et al. Prevention of glucocorticoid-induced osteopenia: effect of oral 25-hydroxyvitamin D and calcium. Clin Rheumatol 1989;8(2):202–7.

[94] Devogelaer JP, Esselinckx W, Nagant de Deuxchaisnes C. Calcidiol protects bone mass in rheumatoid arthritis patients treated by low dose glucocorticoids. In: Norman AW, Bouillon R, Thomasset M, editors. Vitamin D. A pluripotent steroid hormone: structural studies, molecular endocrinology and clinical applications. Berlin: Walter de Gruyter; 1994. p. 855–6.

[95] Talalaj M, Gradowska L, Marcinowska-Suchowierska E, et al. Efficiency of preventive treatment of glucocorticoid-induced osteoporosis with 25-hydroxyvitamin D3 and calcium in kidney transplant patients. Transplant Proc 1996;28(6):3485–7.

[96] Garcia-Delgado I, Prieto S, Gil-Fraguas L, et al. Calcitonin, etidronate, and calcidiol treatment in bone loss after cardiac transplantation. Calcif Tissue Int 1997;60(2):155–9.

[97] Dykman TR, Haralson KM, Gluck OS, et al. Effect of oral 1,25-dihydroxyvitamin D and calcium on glucocorticoid-induced osteopenia in patients with rheumatic diseases. Arthritis Rheum 1984;27(12):1336–43.

[98] Sambrook P, Birmingham J, Kelly P, et al. Prevention of corticosteroid osteoporosis. A comparison of calcium, calcitriol, and calcitonin. N Engl J Med 1993;328(24):1747–52.

[99] Sambrook P, Henderson NK, Keogh A, et al. Effect of calcitriol on bone loss after cardiac or lung transplantation. J Bone Miner Res 2000;15(9):1818–24.

[100] Henderson K, Eisman J, Keogh A, et al. Protective effect of short-term calcitriol or cyclical etidronate on bone loss after cardiac or lung transplantation. J Bone Miner Res 2001;16(3): 565–71.

[101] Braun JJ, Birkenhäger-Frenkel DH, Rietveld AH, et al. Influence of 1α-(OH)D$_3$ administration on bone and bone mineral metabolism in patients on chronic glucocorticoid treatment: a double blind controlled study. Clin Endocrinol (Oxf) 1983;19(2): 265–73.

[102] Reginster JY, Kuntz D, Verdickt W, et al. Prophylactic use of alfacalcidol in corticosteroid-induced osteoporosis. Osteoporos Int 1999;9(1):75–81.

[103] Ringe JD, Cöster A, Meng T, et al. Treatment of glucocorticoid-induced osteoporosis with alfacalcidol/calcium versus vitamin D/calcium. Calcif Tissue Int 1999;65(4):337–40.

[104] Amin S, LaValley MP, Simms RW, et al. The role of vitamin D in corticosteroid-induced osteoporosis: a meta-analytic approach. Arthritis Rheum 1999;42(8):1740–51.

[105] Amin S, Lavalley MP, Simms RW, et al. The comparative efficacy of drug therapies used for the management of corticosteroid-induced osteoporosis: a meta-regression. J Bone Miner Res 2002;17(8):1512–26.

[106] Lukert BP, Johnson BE, Robinson RG. Estrogen and progesterone replacement therapy reduces glucocorticoid-induced bone loss. J Bone Miner Res 1992;7(9):1063–9.

[107] Hall GM, Daniels M, Doyle DV, et al. Effect of hormone replacement therapy on bone mass in rheumatoid arthritis patients treated with and without steroids. Arthritis Rheum 1994;37(10):1499–505.

[108] Writing Group for the Women's Health Initiative Investigators. Risks and benefits of estrogen plus progestin in healthy postmenopausal women. Principal results from the Women's Health Initiative randomized, controlled trial. JAMA 2002;288(3):321–33.

[109] Cummings SR. LIFT study is discontinued. BMJ 2006;332(7542):667.

[110] Fentiman IS, Saad Z, Caleffi M, et al. Tamoxifen protects against steroid-induced bone loss. Eur J Cancer 1992;28(2/3):684–5.

[111] Grecu EO, Weinshelbaum A, Simmons R. Effective therapy of glucocorticoid-induced osteoporosis with medroxyprogesterone acetate. Calcif Tissue Int 1990;46(5):294–9.

[112] Mease PJ, Ginzler EM, Gluck OS, et al. Effects of prasterone on bone mineral density in women with systemic lupus erythematosus receiving chronic glucocorticoid therapy. J Rheumatol 2005;32:616–21.

[113] Cranney A, Welch V, Adachi JD, et al. Calcitonin for preventing and treating corticosteroid-induced osteoporosis (review). The Cochrane Collaboration. The Cochrane Library 2005;1:1–31.

[114] Ringe J-D, Welzel D. Salmon calcitonin in the therapy of corticoid-induced osteoporosis. Eur J Clin Pharmacol 1987;33:35–9.

[115] Böhning W, Ringe JD, Welzel D, et al. Intranasales lachsalcatonin zur prophylaxe des knochenmineral-verkustes bei steroid-bedürftigen chronisch-obstruktiven atemwegserkrankunge. Arzneim-Forsch Drug Res 1990;40(II):1000–3.

[116] Luengo M, Picado C, Del Rio L, et al. Treatment of steroid-induced osteopenia with calcitonin in corticosteroid-dependent asthma. A one-year follow-up study. Am Rev Respir Dis 1990;142:104–7.

[117] Luengo M, Pons F, Martinez de Osaba MJ, et al. Prevention of further bone mass loss by nasal calcitonin in patients on long term glucocorticoid therapy for asthma: a two year follow-up study. Thorax 1994;49(11):1099–102.

[118] Emkey R, Reading W, Procaccini R, the Steroid Induced Osteoporosis Study Group, et al. The effect of calcitonin on bone mass in steroid-induced osteoporosis. Arthritis Rheum 1994;37(Suppl 9):S183.

[119] Healey JH, Paget SA, Williams-Russo P, et al. A randomized controlled trial of salmon calcitonin to prevent bone loss in corticosteroid-treated temporal arteritis and polymyalgia rheumatica. Calcif Tissue Int 1996;58:73–80.

[120] Kotaniemi A, Piirainen H, Paimela L, et al. Is continuous intranasal salmon calcitonin ef-fective in treating axial bone loss in patients with active rheumatoid arthritis receiving low dose glucocorticoid therapy? J Rheumatol 1996;23:1875–9.

[121] Adachi JD, Bensen WG, Bell MJ, et al. Salmon calcitonin nasal spray in the prevention of corticosteroid-induced osteoporosis. Br J Rheumatol 1997;36:255–9.

[122] Mulder H, Struys A. Intermittent cyclical etidronate in the prevention of corticosteroid-induced bone loss. Br J Rheumatol 1994;33:348–50.

[123] Struys A, Snelder AA, Mulder H. Cyclical etidronate reverses bone loss of the spine and proximal femur in patients with established corticosteroid-induced osteoporosis. Am J Med 1995;99(3):235–42.

[124] Van Cleemput J, Daenen W, Geusens P, et al. Prevention of bone loss in cardiac transplant recipients. A comparison of biphosphonates and vitamin D. Transplantation 1996;61: 1495–9.

[125] Adachi JD, Bensen WG, Brown J, et al. Intermittent etidronate therapy to prevent cortico-steroid-induced osteoporosis. N Engl J Med 1997;337:382–7.

[126] Skingle SJ, Moore DJ, Crisp AJ. Cyclical etidronate increases lumbar spine bone density in patients on long-term glucocorticosteroid therapy. Int J Clin Pract 1997;51:364–7.

[127] Wolfhagen FHJ, Van Buuren HR, den Ouden JW, et al. Cyclical etidronate in the preven-tion of bone loss in corticosteroid-treated primary biliary cirrhosis. A prospective, con-trolled pilot study. J Hepatol 1997;26:325–30.

[128] Pitt P, Li F, Todd P, et al. A double blind placebo controlled study to determine the effects of intermittent cyclical etidronate on bone mineral density in patients on long term oral cor-ticosteroid treatment. Thorax 1998;53:351–6.

[129] Roux C, Oriente P, Laan R, et al, for the Ciblos Study Group. Randomized trial of effect of cyclical etidronate in the prevention of corticosteroid-induced bone loss. J Clin Endocrinol Metab 1998;83:1128–33.

[130] Jenkins EA, Walker-Bone KE, Wood A, et al. The prevention of corticosteroid-induced bone loss with intermittent cyclical etidronate. Scand J Rheumatol 1999;28:152–6.

[131] Herrala J, Puolijoki H, Liippo K, et al. Clodronate is effective in preventing corticosteroid-induced bone loss among asthmatic patients. Bone 1998;22(5):577–82.

[132] Frediani B, Falsetti P, Baldi F, et al. Effects of 4-year treatment with once-weekly clodro-nate on prevention of corticosteroid-induced bone loss and fractures in patients with arthri-tis: evaluation with dual-energy X-ray absorptiometry and quantitative ultrasound. Bone 2003;33:575–81.

[133] Boutsen Y, Jamart J, Esselinckx W, Devogelaer JP. Primary prevention of glucocorticoid-induced osteoporosis with intravenous pamidronate and calcium: a prospective controlled 1-year study comparing a single infusion, an infusion given once every 3 months, and cal-cium alone. J Bone Miner Res 2001;16:104–12.

[134] Nzeusseu Toukap A, Depresseux G, Devogelaer JP, et al. Oral pamidronate prevents high-dose glucocorticoid-induced lumbar spine bone loss im premenopausal connective tissue disease (mainly lupus) patients. Lupus 2005;14:517–20.

[135] Saag KG, Emkey R, Schnitzer TJ, et al. Alendronate for the prevention and treatment of glucocorticoid-induced osteoporosis. N Engl J Med 1998;339:292–9.

[136] Eastell R, Devogelaer JP, Peel NFA, et al. Prevention of bone loss with risedronate in glu-cocorticoid-treated rheumatoid arthritis patients. Osteoporos Int 2000;11:331–7.

[137] Shane E, Addesso V, Namerow PB, et al. Alendronate versus calcitriol for the prevention of bone loss after cardiac transplantation. N Engl J Med 2004;350:767–76.

[138] Cohen S, Levy RM, Keller M, et al. Risedronate therapy prevents corticosteroid-induced bone loss. A twelve-month, multicenter, randomized, double-blind, placebo-controlled, parallel-group study. Arthritis Rheum 1999;42:2309–18.

[139] Devogelaer JP, Burckhardt P, Meunier P, et al. Zoledronic acid safety and efficacy over 5 years in post-menopausal osteoporosis. Osteoporos Int 2006;17(Suppl 1):S14.

[140] Rico H, Cabranes JA, Hernandez ER, et al. Reversion of the steroid-induced decrease of serum osteocalcin with sodium fluoride. Clin Rheumatol 1991;10:10–2.

[141] Greenwald M, Brandli D, Spector S, et al. Corticosteroid-induced osteoporosis: effects of a treatment with slow-release sodium fluoride. Osteoporos Int 1992;2:303–4.

[142] Meys E, Terreaux-Duvert F, Beaume-Six T, et al. Bone loss after cardiac transplantation: effects of calcium, calcidiol and monofluorophosphate. Osteoporos Int 1993;3:322–9.

[143] Rizzoli R, Chevalley T, Slosman DO, et al. Sodium monofluorophosphate increases vertebral bone mineral density in patients with corticosteroid-induced osteoporosis. Osteoporos Int 1995;5:39–46.

[144] Guaydier-Souquières G, Kotzki PO, Sabatier JP, et al. In corticosteroid-treated respiratory diseases, monofluorophosphate increases lumbar bone density: a double-masked randomized study. Osteoporos Int 1996;6:171–7.

[145] Lippuner K, Haller B, Casez JP, et al. Effect of disodium monofluorophosphate, calcium and vitamin D supplementation on bone mineral density in patients chronically treated with glucocorticoids: a prospective, randomized, double-blind study. Miner Electrolyte Metab 1996;22:207–13.

[146] Nagant de Deuxchaisnes C, Devogelaer JP. Restorative therapy of osteoporosis. In: Bröll H, Dambacher MA, editors. Osteoporosis: a guide to diagnosis and treatment, Volume 18. Basel (Switzerland): Karger; 1996. p. 207–64.

[147] Lane NE, Sanchez S, Modin GW, et al. Parathyroid hormone treatment can reverse corticosteroid-induced osteoporosis. Results of a randomized controlled clinical trial. J Clin Invest 1998;102:1627–33.

[148] Lane NE, Sanchez S, Modin GW, et al. Bone mass continues to increase at the hip after parathyroid hormone treatment is discontinued in glucocorticoid-induced osteoporosis: results of a randomized controlled clinical trial. J Bone Miner Res 2000;15:944–51.

[149] Buxton EC, Yao W, Lane NE. Changes in serum receptor activator of nuclear factor κBligand, osteoprotegerin, and interleukin-6 levels in patients with glucocorticoid-induced osteoporosis treated with human parathyroid hormone (1–34). J Clin Endocrinol Metab 2004;89(7):3332–6.

[150] Rhen T, Cidlowski JA. Mechanisms of disease. Antiinflammatory action of glucocortioids—new mechanisms for old drugs. N Engl J Med 2005;353(16):1711–23.

[151] Durez PB, Depresseux G, Houssiau FA, Devogelaer J. Follow up of DXA bone mineral density measurement in severe and refractory rheumatoid arthritis (RA) treated with infliximab (IFX). Ann Rheum Dis 2004;63(Suppl 1):96.

[152] Goffin E, Devogelaer JP, Depresseux G, et al. Evaluation of bone mineral density after renal transplantation under a tracolimus-based immunosuppression: a pilot study. Clin Nephrol 2003;59(3):190–5.

RHEUMATIC
DISEASE CLINICS
OF NORTH AMERICA

Rheum Dis Clin N Am 32 (2006) 759–773

Inflammation-Induced Bone Loss: Can it Be Prevented?

Evange Romas, MD, PhD[a],*,
Matthew T. Gillespie, PhD[b]

[a]The University of Melbourne, St. Vincent's Hospital, 41 Victoria Parade,
Fitzroy, 3065, Australia
[b]St. Vincent's Institute, 9 Princes Street, Fitzroy, 3065, Australia

A defining feature of rheumatoid arthritis (RA) is its propensity to destroy cartilage and bone [1]. The presence of bone erosions indicates irreversible joint damage and it is associated with pain, reduced physical and emotional functioning, and increased mortality [2]. Arthritic bone destruction is associated with systemic osteoporosis and susceptibility to fragility fractures, because both phenomena reflect high inflammatory disease activity [3,4].

Osteoclasts (OCLs) are cells that are uniquely capable of bone degradation, and the concept that OCLs drive bone loss in RA is now accepted widely [5]. OCLs are consistently detected at erosion sites in all animal models of destructive arthritis as well as human RA [6]. Synovial inflammation generates tumor necrosis factor (TNF)-α, macrophage colony-stimulating factor (M-CSF), and receptor activator of nuclear factor-κB ligand (RANKL)—cytokines that fuel osteoclastogenesis and arthritic bone destruction. The targeted removal of OCLs by TNF blockers, RANKL antagonism, or genetic manipulation in animal models potently blocks this bone destruction [7–12].

The bone loss in RA is a consequence of distorted bone remodeling in the context of chronic inflammation. OCLs and osteoblasts are present near active bone erosions, and it is likely that defects of both cell types contribute to the bone loss. Although OCLs are abundant and highly activated, simultaneously the osteoblasts are suppressed by exposure to inflammatory cytokines (eg, TNF) [13]. The importance of osteoclasts has prompted renewed interest

---

* Corresponding author.
E-mail address: romase@svhm.org.au (E. Romas).

0889-857X/06/$ - see front matter © 2006 Elsevier Inc. All rights reserved.
doi:10.1016/j.rdc.2006.07.004   *rheumatic.theclinics.com*

in bisphosphonates (BPs) to address inflammatory bone loss. In fact, targeting OCLs with powerful BPs confers bone protection in autoimmune or TNF-dependent models of RA [14,15]. Down-regulation of OCLs has emerged as a powerful strategy for prevention of inflammation-induced bone loss. Significantly, the bone protection that is afforded by OCL down-regulation is not always conditional on reduced synovial inflammation.

For clinicians, the prevention of structural joint damage is now a central tenet of contemporary antirheumatic drug therapy [16]. A concerted approach to address inflammatory bone loss requires consideration of several possible strategies: (1) intensive interference with inflammatory synovial processes that stimulate bone erosion, and most of all, overproduction of TNF-α; (2) blockade of pathogenic OCLs; and (3) increased osteoblast recruitment or osteoblast function to promote skeletal repair.

Bone loss in rheumatoid arthritis

Three distinct types of bone loss are delineated in RA: focal articular bone erosion, juxta-articular osteopenia adjacent to arthritis, and systemic osteoporosis at sites distant from inflamed joints. Radiographic bone erosions are associated highly with systemic osteoporosis [17], because both phenomena are linked fundamentally to persistently high disease activity.

Erosive RA is characterized by the presence of autoantibodies to IgG (rheumatoid factors) and cyclic citrullinated peptides [18,19]. MRI may detect erosions in up to 70% of patients who have RA after only 6 months [20]. MRI detects increased proton density in the bone marrow adjacent to inflamed joints—in the absence and presence of bone erosions. The histologic correlate of the "bone marrow edema" is not well defined; however, aspiration has yielded hemopoietic CD34$^+$ bone marrow cells that are potential OCL precursors [21].

Juxta-articular osteopenia that is adjacent to inflamed joints is one of the first radiographic signs of RA, maximal in early disease, correlates positively with disease activity and negatively with disease duration. Biopsies of juxta-articular bone have revealed numerous OCLs as well as increased osteoid and resorptive surfaces that are consistent with high bone turnover and negative bone balance [22].

Generalized osteoporosis is prevalent in RA and is associated with increased fracture rates. Unlike postmenopausal osteoporosis, osteoporosis in RA is characterized by relatively preserved axial (lumbar spine) bone and marked loss at appendicular sites (hip and radius). The main determinant of systemic bone loss is the underlying inflammatory disease process. Thus, higher bone loss in early RA (assessed by bone densitometry or biomarkers of osteoclastic activity) is correlated with measures of higher disease activity (serum C-reactive protein) [23].

Osteoclastogenesis and arthritic bone destruction

RANKL is a TNF family cytokine that is essential for induction of osteoclastogenesis. This function was revealed by targeted disruption of the gene in mice, which resulted in defective lymph node organogenesis and lymphocyte differentiation, and osteopetrosis caused by a complete absence of OCLs [24]. Therefore, the discovery of the RANKL/RANK/osteoprotegerin (OPG) system defined the central molecular basis of osteoclastogenesis, and revealed the nexus between the immune system and bone in RA [24,25].

After the discovery that osteoclastogenesis and bone turnover were regulated by expression of RANKL/RANK and its soluble decoy receptor, OPG, their expression was investigated in arthritis. These studies revealed that RANKL mRNA was detected by reverse transcriptase–polymerase chain reaction in synovium from RA but not from healthy synovium [26]. RANKL has been detected in synovial fibroblasts and activated T cells from peripheral blood as well as tissue near the pannus–bone interface [27–29]. In the authors' in situ hybridization studies, CD3+ T cells, osteoblasts, and fibroblast-like synoviocytes in RA synovium all stained intensely for RANKL [28]. Similarly, in collagen-induced arthritis (CIA), RANKL and OPG were detected at the erosion sites [12].

OCL-mediated joint destruction also was delineated in psoriatic arthritis (PsA), which, like RA, is characterized by intense synovitis and bone destruction [30]. The severity of bone erosion was correlated to higher circulating mononuclear OCL precursor (OcP) numbers, which revealed a novel mechanism for osteoclastogenesis in PsA [30]. Circulating OcPs also were elevated in human TNF transgenic (hTNF Tg) mice, and OcP numbers decreased after anti-TNF therapy [31]. Recently, it was shown that TNF-α increases the number of circulating OcPs by promoting their proliferation and differentiation in the bone marrow through up-regulation of the M-CSF receptor, c-*fms* [32].

In vitro studies showed that osteoblasts and T cells expressed RANKL and supported OCL differentiation when cocultured with myeloid precursors [25,28,33]. Cocultures of synovial fibroblasts and monocytes also generated OCLs in vitro [27]. Hence, multiple cell types that are present in inflamed synovium, such as activated T cells, fibroblasts, and osteoblastic stromal cells, express RANKL.

OCL formation in arthritis models is a swift and dynamic process that leads to rapid attack on juxta-articular bone, a prerequisite for early-onset structural damage [34,35]. Because OCLs have a finite life span, continuous replenishment of local OCL pools probably is necessary to achieve progressive bone damage [36]. From the perspective of bone erosions in RA, major cellular targets of RANKL are RANK-positive OcPs, primarily monocytes that populate inflamed synovium, as well as myeloid lineage cells resident in bone marrow. Direct cell-to-cell contact between stromal cells and OcPs efficiently presents the required molecular signals (ie, RANKL + M-CSF) for OCL differentiation (Fig. 1) [37]. At the pannus–bone interface, the main stromal OCL support cells are the fibroblast-like synoviocytes, whereas the major OCL support cells in subchondral bone are osteoblasts.

The role of T cells in inflammation-induced bone loss

Although T cells express RANKL, they also produce OCL inhibitors, such as interferon (IFN)-γ and interleukin (IL)-4 [38–40]. IFN-β production that is induced by RANKL autoregulates osteoclastogenesis [41]. Thus, the actual role of T cells in osteoclastogenesis is highly complex and may depend on the suite of prevailing cytokines [42]. Under some conditions, T cells may not drive osteoclastogenesis, even if RANKL is expressed. In the presence of high levels of TNF, subosteoclastogenic ("permissive") amounts of RANKL may be sufficient for TNF to drive RANKL-mediated osteoclastogenesis [43]. In essence, although there is a potential contribution of soluble RANKL from T cells, expression of membrane RANKL by fibroblast-like synoviocytes or osteoblasts (induced by factors, such as IL-6–type cytokines or IL-17) may be more importantly quantitatively for osteoclastogenesis in the inflamed joint [44,45].

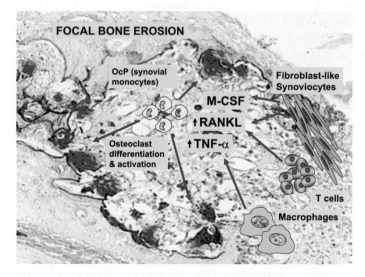

Fig. 1. Cellular and molecular interactions in the synovial compartment that elicit OCL-mediated bone erosions in RA. Synovial monocytes constitute OCL precursor cells. The predominant stromal support cells are activated fibroblast-like synoviocytes that express M-CSF as well as RANKL. The high levels of TNF-α (secreted by synovial macrophages) promote massive osteoclastogenesis in the context of RANKL. OCLs are the dark red cells adjacent to resorption pits. RANKL also activates and extends the life span of nascent osteoclasts.

Transcriptional control of osteoclastogenesis

The transcriptional program that controls osteoclastogenesis is highly intricate. OCL differentiation depends on RANK and immunoreceptor tyrosine-based activation motif (ITAM) signals in OCL precursors [46]. The phosphorylation of ITAM stimulated by immunoreceptors and RANKL–RANK interaction results in the recruitment of Syk family kinases. This leads to the activation of phospholipase Cγ and calcium signaling, which is critical for the nuclear factor of activated T cells c1 (NFATc1) induction, a master transcription factor for OCL development [47]. NFATc1 induction also is dependent on c-Fos and TNF receptor-associated factor 6, which are activated by RANKL [48,49]. Mice that are deficient in the DNAX-activating protein (DAP)12 and FcRγ ITAM-bearing adapters are osteopetrotic with a severe defect in OCL differentiation, which demonstrates the requirement for ITAM signals in bone [46,50,51]. ITAM signals that are mediated through FcRγ are activated by ligands that are expressed by osteoblasts, whereas those that are associated with DAP12 are activated by ligands that are expressed on OCL precursors themselves [52]. Their regulation by ITAM-dependent receptors implies that OCLs are controlled tightly by arrays of receptors that confer responsiveness to their local microenvironment, like innate immune cells.

Targeting tumor necrosis factor α to prevent arthritic bone destruction

RA is a persistent and symmetric polyarthritis that affects the metacarpophalangeal and proximal interphalangeal joints of the hands and small joints of feet, as well as wrists, elbows, shoulders, knees, and ankles. The synovitis in RA is accompanied by intense neovascularization. Egress of inflammatory cells and local cellular proliferation together result in marked synovial expansion, which creates numerous synovial villi that protrude into the joint space. The proliferated synovium forms a tissue (pannus) that lies in direct contact with the articular surface. Histologically, RA synovium is characterized by hyperplasia of synovial lining cells and infiltration of the sublining layer by lymphocytes, activated macrophages, plasma cells, and other cell types. Inflammatory mediators that are released by cells resident in the synovium and pannus contribute to joint destruction. Also, variable bone marrow inflammation recently was identified in RA, although its importance for driving bone erosion is unknown [53,54].

The inflamed synovium is an exceptional source of inflammatory cytokines, such as TNF-α, IL-1, IL-6, and IL-17 [55]. All of these cytokines increase the stromal cell expression of RANKL or reduce OPG expression. Through pleiotropic activities on multiple cells TNF-α is the dominant cytokine for arthritic bone destruction. The high TNF production probably is responsible for endowing the rheumatoid synovium with its proclivity for bone destruction. Unlike benign arthropathies, RA is characterized by greater synovial TNF induction and higher levels of TNF in the synovial fluids [56], which preferentially promotes osteoclastogenesis through the p55 receptor on OCL progenitors [57]. TNF production is stimulated by T-cell–derived IFN-γ and direct cell-to-cell contact of macrophages with T cells [58,59]. The immunogenetic susceptibility that is conferred by the presence of the "shared epitope" is associated with production of rheumatoid factor (RF) and anti–cyclic citrullinated peptides; the resultant immune complexes amplify monocyte/macrophage TNF production in the joints [60].

Specific actions of TNF to promote osteoclastogenesis are: (1) TNF directly promotes OCL differentiation of monocytes and macrophages exposed to RANKL [8]; (2) TNF stimulates stromal-osteoblast RANKL production (through a mechanism involving IL-1 and IL-17) [61]; (3) TNF stimulates RANKL production by T and B cells; (4) TNF stimulates stromal-osteoblast production of M-CSF [62]; and (5) TNF enhances stromal cell expression of RANKL [55].

Remarkably, the TNF blockers in clinical use tend to interfere more consistently with joint destruction than with inflammatory synovitis. In some patients, TNF antagonism may arrest structural joint damage despite little improvement in inflammation [63]. The "disconnect" between bone destruction and inflammation may imply that TNF is a principal driver for bone loss, whereas other cytokines are responsible for symptoms. Alternatively, TNF levels may be reduced to subthreshold levels such that OCL generation is suppressed, while sufficient TNF is available to mediate synovial inflammation.

Besides TNF, the other key inflammatory cytokines are IL-1 and IL-6. The involvement of these cytokines is supported by the occurrence of erosive arthritis in mice that lack the IL-1 receptor antagonist (IL-1ra) and inhibitory effects of IL-6 receptor antibodies in experimental arthritis [64–66]. Overall, IL-1 antagonism is not as efficacious as is TNF blockade to prevent bone erosions in RA [67]. Although this may reflect suboptimal dosing of IL-1ra, more likely (although this premise is controversial) it implies a lesser role for IL-1 [68]. With respect to OCL biology, TNF drives OCL differentiation (through p55 receptors), whereas IL-1 is more important for extending the life span of nascent OCLs [10]. Evidently, a destructive synergy may exist between TNF, IL-17, IL-1, and the IL-6 type cytokines, to induce RANK-mediated bone loss [55].

In contrast to successful TNF blockade, measurable joint damage continues in many patients who are treated with traditional disease-modifying drugs (eg, methotrexate [MTX]), although at a much reduced rate. This suggests that continuing TNF production is sufficient to stimulate osteoclastic erosion in many patients who are treated with MTX. Actually, MTX therapy may reduce endogenous IL-1 preferentially, which may explain the greater clinical benefits (for radiologic progression) of adding TNF blockers to MTX [69–71].

Targeting osteoclastogenesis

Proof of the role of OCLs in inflammatory bone loss came from models of arthritis and especially by using genetically altered mice. In initial studies, OPG prevented articular bone destruction in adjuvant arthritis and CIA [12,25]. Similarly, mutant mice that completely lacked OCLs (RANKL-deficient or *c-fos*–deficient mice) were protected from arthritic bone destruction that was induced by serum transfer (from K/BxN Tg mice) or by crossing them with hTNF Tg mice [8,11]. TNF-mediated bone loss (in the hTNF Tg mice) was reduced effectively by treatment with Fc-OPG or RANK:Fc or by crossing with RANK$^{-/-}$ mutants, as well as by the TNF antibody infliximab [7,9,72].

In all models, drastically reduced OCL numbers were associated with bone protection, yet synovial inflammation was not reduced by RANKL antagonism. Notably, cartilage protection in these models was minimal or absent. This confirmed the view that divergent cellular mechanisms are responsible for bone or cartilage loss [55,73], because cartilage damage largely is independent of RANK-mediated osteoclastogenesis. These findings are consistent with the involvement of a disintegrin and metalloprotease with thrombospondin motifs (ADAM-TS)5 in arthritic cartilage degradation [74,75].

The prospects for anti-RANKL therapy were reviewed recently [76]. OPG or peptide mimetics of OPG effectively prevent OCL-mediated bone destruction in diverse animal models; however, Fc-OPG protein rapidly elicits neutralizing antibodies that limit its utility. The therapeutic potential of RANKL monoclonal antibodies (eg, Denosumab) was reported in postmenopausal women who had osteoporosis. Single subcutaneous injections of Denosumab reduced biomarkers of bone resorption for up to 6 months in a dose-dependent fashion [77,78]. Other investigators reported the usefulness of a RANKL vaccine in preventing arthritic joint destruction in mice [79]. Approaches that target the intracellular RANK signaling cascade are interesting, but have to circumvent the key issues of drug delivery and cell and tissue specificity [76]. Monoclonal antibodies that neutralize RANKL are the most promising candidate for anti-RANKL therapy.

Bisphosphonates for inflammation-induced bone loss

BPs are analogs of inorganic pyrophosphate in which an oxygen atom has been replaced with a carbon atom. The phosphate–carbon–phosphate moiety confers a high-affinity binding to solid-phase calcium phosphate where the drugs preferentially interfere with osteoclastic bone resorption. Their properties have been reviewed extensively [80,81]. The more potent amino-BPs alendronate, risedronate, ibandronate, and zoledronate exert their inhibitory effects on OCL function by inhibiting farnesyl pyrophosphate synthase, an enzyme in the mevalonate pathway that is necessary for lipid modification (prenylation) of small GTP-binding proteins. This process alters cytoskeletal organization and intracellular trafficking that result in inhibition of OCL function. The nonamino-BPs (eg, etidronate and clodronate) are metabolized to nonhydrolyzable analogs of ATP, and act as inhibitors of ATP-dependent enzymes, which leads to enhanced OCL apoptosis.

Based on the insights that were gained from targeting RANKL in arthritis, invoking BPs for bone protection in RA is logical; however, the use of BPs in arthritis is not a novel idea. The first- and second-generation BPs were tested in arthritis models, primarily as anti-inflammatory drugs that targeted macrophages. These early studies reported reduced biomarkers of bone resorption and variable joint protection; however, any effects on focal bone erosion were documented poorly [82–85].

The authors reported a quantitative analysis of the effect of zoledronic acid (ZA), a highly potent BP, on bone and joint structure in CIA [15]. A single pulse of ZA effectively prevented radiologic bone erosions in this arthritis model (Fig. 2). At the highest dose then tested (100 μg/kg) histologic

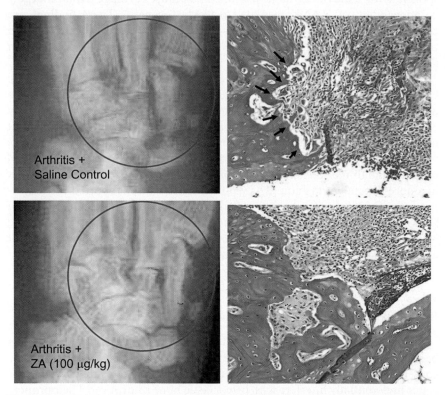

Fig. 2. Radiologic bone erosions are prevented by ZA. CIA treated at its onset without (*top panel*) or with (*lower panel*) a single injection of ZA, 100 μg/kg. The arthritic joints were radiographed and processed for histology after 2 weeks. The right upper panel shows numerous osteoclastic erosion sites (*arrows*) in arthritic joints from untreated animals, which are prevented by ZA given at the onset of arthritis (*right lower panel*).

erosion scores were reduced by 80%. Juxta-articular bone loss was prevented, trabecular bone mass increased to greater than control levels, and the elevated bone resorption biomarker C-telopeptide of collagen type-1 was normalized. In contrast, ZA had no useful effect on synovitis or cartilage damage. Larger dosages of ZA (50–100 µg/kg) had a mildly proinflammatory effect, and, despite the continuing synovitis, ZA protected arthritic bone. A study that used repetitive dosing of ZA in the TNF Tg mice showed comparable reduction in bone erosions and prevention of systemic osteoporosis [14]. OCL numbers in both studies were reduced drastically. From the authors' detailed histomorphometric analysis it is concluded that ZA exerted bone protection by down-regulating OCL numbers as well as by reducing OCL activity [15]. In contrast, the authors have observed that salmon calcitonin, a weaker antiresorptive agent that does not down-regulate OCL numbers, failed to modulate bone erosions in CIA (unpublished data).

It is uncertain whether BPs could inhibit radiologic bone erosion in RA and this issue was reviewed recently [86]. Short-term MRI studies suggest that the protective effects of ZA could be recapitulated in RA [87]. The most potent third-generation BPs that exhibit the most profound inhibitory effects on OCLs have not been assessed in sufficiently powered controlled trials with radiologic erosion as a primary end point. Because up to 40% of patients do not respond to TNF antagonists, and as a result of their high costs and uncertain long-term safety, investigations of the third-generation BPs to prevent inflammatory-induced bone loss in RA are necessary and rational.

Targeting osteoblasts to reverse inflammatory bone loss

It is unknown if RA bone erosions can be reconstituted properly, although reports of erosion "repair" after anti-inflammatory therapy are testament to this possibility [88]. Osteoclastic activity cannot be viewed separately from osteoblasts because these two cell populations are linked through physiologic coupling [89]. Osteoblasts are present in bone erosions; however, the detailed kinetics and fate of osteoblasts relative to OCLs at erosion sites has not been elucidated [53]. In view of the coupling of osteoblasts to OCLs, it is likely that osteoblasts at erosion sites are recruited as a response to osteoclastic activity, not reactive to inflammatory synovitis, although this has not been resolved. Clearly, the osteoblastic response in active erosions is feeble, and results in net bone loss. Cytokines, such as TNF, down-regulate osteoblasts, in part by interfering with the master transcription factor Runx-2 [13,90,91]. Fundamentally, osteoblastic suppression in arthritis may be additive to the bone-damaging effects of TNF-induced osteoclastogenesis.

Parathyroid hormone (PTH) is the only useful bone anabolic agent available; its use has been documented extensively in animals and humans who have osteoporosis after estrogen deficiency [92]. The effects of PTH are governed by the dynamics of its presentation to osteoblasts. At a constant level, PTH down-regulates OPG, which increases osteoclastogenesis, whereas pulsed administration also stimulates osteoblastogenesis, increases bone remodeling, and leads to gains in bone mass. Pulsed PTH therapy was tested in animal models of inflammatory bone loss. Short-term PTH alone had no measurable effects on bone destruction in the hTNF Tg mice; however, together with anti-TNF or anti-RANKL therapy, mice that were treated with PTH exhibited greater bone protection and repair of articular erosions [93]. Similar effects were reported in immune-mediated models of arthritis [94]; however, concomitant OCL inhibition may blunt the effect of PTH in humans, as was reported with alendronate [89,95]. Therefore, it remains to be seen if these results could be reproduced clinically in settings that require profound OCL inhibition.

Summary

Inflammatory synovitis induces profound bone loss and OCLs are the instrument of this destruction. TNF blockers have an established role in the prevention of inflammatory bone loss in RA; however, not all patients respond to anti-TNF therapy and side effects may prevent long-term treatment in others. The B-cell–depleting antibody rituximab and the T-cell costimulation blocker abatacept are emerging as major treatment options for patients who are resistant to anti-TNF [96,97]. Proof-of-concept studies demonstrate that targeting RANK-mediated osteoclastogenesis prevents inflammatory bone loss and clinical application has only just begun. The efficacy of RANKL inhibition has been witnessed in trials of Denosumab, and RANKL-neutralizing antibodies are likely to become the treatment of choice for blocking RANKL in RA [77,78]. A major limitation of RANKL antagonism is that it does not treat synovitis. Therefore, anti-RANKL therapy most likely will be used in the context of MTX therapy. There is uncertainty about the possible extraskeletal adverse effects of long-term RANKL blockade. In particular, anti-RANKL therapy could jeopardize dendritic cell function or survival. The demonstrable role of OCLs in inflammation-induced bone loss also invites a reconsideration of the new BPs for bone protection [98]. Studies of ZA in preclinical models indicate that bone protection is comparable to that afforded by OPG. One possible caveat is that intravenous BPs are linked to jaw osteonecrosis [99], although the incidence is confined mainly to intensive treatment in the oncology setting. Although pulsed PTH stimulated bone formation in arthritic models, it has yet to be proven clinically in the context of powerful OCL inhibition with TNF or RANKL antagonists. With strategies that normalize OCL numbers, clinicians are poised to accomplish effective prevention of inflammation-induced bone loss.

Acknowledgments

This work was funded by grant support from the NHMRC (Australia).

References

[1] Goldring S. Osteoporosis and rheumatic diseases. In: Favus MJ, editor. Primer of the metabolic bone diseases and disorders of mineral metabolism. 5th edition. Philadelphia: Lippincott Williams & Wilkins; 2003. p. 379–82.

[2] Drossaers-Bakker KW, de Buck M, van Zeben D, et al. Long-term course and outcome of functional capacity in rheumatoid arthritis: the effect of disease activity and radiologic damage over time. Arthritis Rheum 1999;42(9):1854–60.

[3] Forsblad D'Elia H, Larsen A, Waltbrand E, et al. Radiographic joint destruction in post-menopausal rheumatoid arthritis is strongly associated with generalised osteoporosis. Ann Rheum Dis 2003;62(7):617–23.

[4] Gough AK, Lilley J, Eyre S, et al. Generalised bone loss in patients with early rheumatoid arthritis. Lancet 1994;344(8914):23–7.

[5] Goldring SR. Pathogenesis of bone and cartilage destruction in rheumatoid arthritis. Rheumatology (Oxford) 2003;42(Suppl 2):ii11–6.

[6] Gravallese EM, Harada Y, Wang JT, et al. Identification of cell types responsible for bone resorption in rheumatoid arthritis and juvenile rheumatoid arthritis. Am J Pathol 1998; 152(4):943–51.

[7] Redlich K, Hayer S, Maier A, et al. Tumor necrosis factor alpha-mediated joint destruction is inhibited by targeting osteoclasts with osteoprotegerin. Arthritis Rheum 2002;46(3): 785–92.

[8] Redlich K, Hayer S, Ricci R, et al. Osteoclasts are essential for TNF alpha mediated joint destruction. J Clin Invest 2002;110(10):1419–27.

[9] Schett G, Redlich K, Hayer S, et al. Osteoprotegerin protects against generalized bone loss in tumor necrosis factor-transgenic mice. Arthritis Rheum 2003;48(7):2042–51.

[10] Zwerina J, Hayer S, Tohidast-Akrad M, et al. Single and combined inhibition of tumor necrosis factor, interleukin-1, and RANKL pathways in tumor necrosis factor-induced arthritis: effects on synovial inflammation, bone erosion, and cartilage destruction. Arthritis Rheum 2004;50(1):277–90.

[11] Pettit AR, Ji H, von Stechow D, et al. TRANCE/RANKL knockout mice are protected from bone erosion in a serum transfer model of arthritis. Am J Pathol 2001;159(5):1689–99.

[12] Romas E, Sims NA, Hards DK, et al. Osteoprotegerin reduces osteoclast numbers and prevents bone erosion in collagen-induced arthritis. Am J Pathol 2002;161(4): 1419–27.

[13] Bertolini DR, Nedwin GE, Bringman TS, et al. Stimulation of bone resorption and inhibition of bone formation in vitro by human tumour necrosis factors. Nature 1986;319(6053): 516–8.

[14] Herrak P, Gortz B, Hayer S, et al. Zoledronic acid protects against local and systemic bone loss in tumor necrosis factor-mediated arthritis. Arthritis Rheum 2004;50(7): 2327–37.

[15] Sims NA, Green JR, Glatt M, et al. Targeting osteoclasts with zoledronic acid prevents bone destruction in collagen-induced arthritis. Arthritis Rheum 2004;50(7):2338–46.

[16] Smolen JS, Steiner G. Therapeutic strategies for rheumatoid arthritis. Nat Rev Drug Discov 2003;2(6):473–88.

[17] Sambrook PN. The skeleton in rheumatoid arthritis: common mechanisms for bone erosion and osteoporosis? J Rheumatol 2000;27(11):2541–2.

[18] Vincent C, Nogueira L, Clavel C, et al. Autoantibodies to citrullinated proteins: ACPA. Autoimmunity 2005;38(1):17–24.

[19] Cappellen D, Luong-Nguyen NH, Bongiovanni S, et al. Transcriptional program of mouse osteoclast differentiation governed by the macrophage colony-stimulating factor and the ligand for the receptor activator of NFkappa B. J Biol Chem 2002;277(24):21971–82.

[20] Ostergaard M, Hansen M, Stoltenberg M, et al. New radiographic bone erosions in the wrists of patients with rheumatoid arthritis are detectable with magnetic resonance imaging a median of two years earlier. Arthritis Rheum 2003;48(8):2128–31.

[21] Mc Gonagle D, Gibbon W, O'Connor P, et al. A preliminary study of ultrasound aspiration of bone erosion in early rheumatoid arthritis. Rheumatology (Oxford) 1999;38(4):329–31.

[22] Shimizu S, Shiozawa S, Shiozawa K, et al. Quantitative histologic studies on the pathogenesis of periarticular osteoporosis in rheumatoid arthritis. Arthritis Rheum 1985;28(1):25–31.

[23] Gough A, Sambrook P, Devlin J, et al. Osteoclastic activation is the principal mechanism leading to secondary osteoporosis in rheumatoid arthritis. J Rheumatol 1998;25(7):1282–9.

[24] Kong YY, Yoshida H, Sarosi I, et al. OPGL is a key regulator of osteoclastogenesis, lymphocyte development and lymph-node organogenesis. Nature 1999;397(6717):315–23.

[25] Kong YY, Feige U, Sarosi I, et al. Activated T cells regulate bone loss and joint destruction in adjuvant arthritis through osteoprotegerin ligand. Nature 1999;402(6759):304–9.

[26] Gravallese EM, Manning C, Tsay A, et al. Synovial tissue in rheumatoid arthritis is a source of osteoclast differentiation factor. Arthritis Rheum 2000;43(2):250–8.

[27] Takayanagi H, Iizuka H, Juji T, et al. Involvement of receptor activator of nuclear factor kappaB ligand/osteoclast differentiation factor in osteoclastogenesis from synoviocytes in rheumatoid arthritis. Arthritis Rheum 2000;43(2):259–69.

[28] Horwood NJ, Kartsogiannis V, Quinn JM, et al. Activated T lymphocytes support osteoclast formation in vitro. Biochem Biophys Res Commun 1999;265(1):144–50.

[29] Pettit AR, Walsh NC, Manning C, et al. RANKL protein is expressed at the pannus-bone interface at sites of articular bone erosion in rheumatoid arthritis. Rheumatology (Oxford) 2006;45(9):1068–76.

[30] Ritchlin CT, Haas-Smith SA, Li P, et al. Mechanisms of TNF-alpha- and RANKL-mediated osteoclastogenesis and bone resorption in psoriatic arthritis. J Clin Invest 2003;111(6): 821–31.

[31] Li P, Schwarz EM, O'Keefe RJ, et al. Systemic tumor necrosis factor alpha mediates an increase in peripheral CD11bhigh osteoclast precursors in tumor necrosis factor alpha-transgenic mice. Arthritis Rheum 2004;50(1):265–76.

[32] Yao Z, Li P, Zhang Q, et al. TNF increases circulating osteoclast precursor numbers by promoting their proliferation and differentiation in the bone marrow through up-regulation of c-fms expression. J Biol Chem 2006;281(17):11846–55.

[33] Shigeyama Y, Pap T, Kunzler P, et al. Expression of osteoclast differentiation factor in rheumatoid arthritis. Arthritis Rheum 2000;43(11):2523–30.

[34] Lubberts E, Oppers-Walgreen B, Pettit AR, et al. Increase in expression of receptor activator of nuclear factor kappaB at sites of bone erosion correlates with progression of inflammation in evolving collagen-induced arthritis. Arthritis Rheum 2002;46(11):3055–64.

[35] Schett G, Stolina M, Bolon B, et al. Analysis of the kinetics of osteoclastogenesis in arthritic rats. Arthritis Rheum 2005;52(10):3192–201.

[36] Teitelbaum SL. Bone resorption by osteoclasts. Science 2000;289(5484):1504–8.

[37] Suda T, Takahashi N, Udagawa N, et al. Modulation of osteoclast differentiation and function by the new members of the tumor necrosis factor receptor and ligand families. Endocr Rev 1999;20(3):345–57.

[38] Fox SW, Chambers TJ. Interferon-gamma directly inhibits TRANCE-induced osteoclastogenesis. Biochem Biophys Res Commun 2000;276(3):868–72.

[39] Wei S, Wang MW, Teitelbaum SL, et al. Interleukin-4 reversibly inhibits osteoclastogenesis via inhibition of NF-kappa B and mitogen-activated protein kinase signaling. J Biol Chem 2002;277(8):6622–30.

[40] Takayanagi H, Ogasawara K, Hida S, et al. T-cell-mediated regulation of osteoclastogenesis by signalling cross-talk between RANKL and IFN-gamma. Nature 2000;408(6812):600–5.

[41] Takayanagi H, Kim S, Matsuo K, et al. RANKL maintains bone homeostasis through c-Fos-dependent induction of interferon-beta. Nature 2002;416(6882):744–9.

[42] Wyzga N, Varghese S, Wikel S, et al. Effects of activated T cells on osteoclastogenesis depend on how they are activated. Bone 2004;35(3):614–20.

[43] Lam J, Takeshita S, Barker JE, et al. TNF-alpha induces osteoclastogenesis by direct stimulation of macrophages exposed to permissive levels of RANK ligand. J Clin Invest 2000; 106(12):1481–8.

[44] Kotake S, Udagawa N, Takahashi N, et al. IL-17 in synovial fluids from patients with rheumatoid arthritis is a potent stimulator of osteoclastogenesis. J Clin Invest 1999;103(9): 1345–52.

[45] Palmqvist P, Persson E, Conaway HH, et al. IL-6, leukemia inhibitory factor, and oncostatin M stimulate bone resorption and regulate the expression of receptor activator of NF-kappa B ligand, osteoprotegerin, and receptor activator of NF-kappa B in mouse calvariae. J Immunol 2002;169(6):3353–62.

[46] Koga T, Inui M, Inoue K, et al. Costimulatory signals mediated by the ITAM motif cooperate with RANKL for bone homeostasis. Nature 2004;428(6984):758–63.

[47] Takayanagi H, Kim S, Koga T, et al. Induction and activation of the transcription factor NFATc1 (NFAT2) integrate RANKL signaling in terminal differentiation of osteoclasts. Dev Cell 2002;3(6):889–901.

[48] Matsuo K, Galson DL, Zhao C, et al. Nuclear factor of activated T-cells (NFAT) rescues osteoclastogenesis in precursors lacking c-Fos. J Biol Chem 2004;279(25):26475–80.

[49] Gohda J, Akiyama T, Koga T, et al. RANK-mediated amplification of TRAF6 signaling leads to NFATc1 induction during osteoclastogenesis. EMBO J 2005;24(4):790–9.

[50] Kaifu T, Nakahara J, Inui M, et al. Osteopetrosis and thalamic hypomyelinosis with synaptic degeneration in DAP12-deficient mice. J Clin Invest 2003;111(3):323–32.

[51] Mocsai A, Humphrey MB, Van Ziffle JA, et al. The immunomodulatory adapter proteins DAP12 and Fc receptor gamma-chain (FcRgamma) regulate development of functional osteoclasts through the Syk tyrosine kinase. Proc Natl Acad Sci U S A 2004;101(16): 6158–63.

[52] Takayanagi H. Mechanistic insight into osteoclast differentiation in osteoimmunology. J Mol Med 2005;83(3):170–9.

[53] Jimenez-Boj E, Redlich K, Turk B, et al. Interaction between synovial inflammatory tissue and bone marrow in rheumatoid arthritis. J Immunol 2005;175(4):2579–88.

[54] Bugatti S, Caporali R, Manzo A, et al. Involvement of subchondral bone marrow in rheumatoid arthritis: lymphoid neogenesis and in situ relationship to subchondral bone marrow osteoclast recruitment. Arthritis Rheum 2005;52(11):3448–59.

[55] Romas E, Gillespie MT, Martin TJ. Involvement of receptor activator of NFkappaB ligand and tumor necrosis factor-alpha in bone destruction in rheumatoid arthritis. Bone 2002; 30(2):340–6.

[56] Partsch G, Steiner G, Leeb BF, et al. Highly increased levels of tumor necrosis factor-alpha and other proinflammatory cytokines in psoriatic arthritis synovial fluid. J Rheumatol 1997; 24(3):518–23.

[57] Abu-Amer Y, Ross FP, Edwards J, et al. Lipopolysaccharide-stimulated osteoclastogenesis is mediated by tumor necrosis factor via its P55 receptor. J Clin Invest 1997;100(6):1557–65.

[58] McInnes IB, Leung BP, Sturrock RD, et al. Interleukin-15 mediates T cell-dependent regulation of tumor necrosis factor-alpha production in rheumatoid arthritis. Nat Med 1997; 3(2):189–95.

[59] Koerner TJ, Adams DO, Hamilton TA. Regulation of tumor necrosis factor (TNF) expression: interferon-gamma enhances the accumulation of mRNA for TNF induced by lipopolysaccharide in murine peritoneal macrophages. Cell Immunol 1987;109(2):437–43.

[60] Debets JM, Van der Linden CJ, Dieteren IE, et al. Fc-receptor cross-linking induces rapid secretion of tumor necrosis factor (cachectin) by human peripheral blood monocytes. J Immunol 1988;141(4):1197–201.

[61] Wei S, Kitaura H, Zhou P, et al. IL-1 mediates TNF-induced osteoclastogenesis. J Clin Invest 2005;115(2):282–90.
[62] Kitaura H, Zhou P, Kim HJ, et al. M-CSF mediates TNF-induced inflammatory osteolysis. J Clin Invest 2005;115(12):3418–27.
[63] Smolen JS, Han C, Bala M, et al. Evidence of radiographic benefit of treatment with infliximab plus methotrexate in rheumatoid arthritis patients who had no clinical improvement: a detailed subanalysis of data from the anti-tumor necrosis factor trial in rheumatoid arthritis with concomitant therapy study. Arthritis Rheum 2005;52(4):1020–30.
[64] Nakae S, Saijo S, Horai R, et al. IL-17 production from activated T cells is required for the spontaneous development of destructive arthritis in mice deficient in IL-1 receptor antagonist. Proc Natl Acad Sci U S A 2003;100(10):5986–90.
[65] Takagi N, Mihara M, Moriya Y, et al. Blockage of interleukin-6 receptor ameliorates joint disease in murine collagen-induced arthritis. Arthritis Rheum 1998;41(12):2117–21.
[66] Wong PK, Quinn JM, Sims NA, et al. Interleukin-6 modulates production of T lymphocyte-derived cytokines in antigen-induced arthritis and drives inflammation-induced osteoclastogenesis. Arthritis Rheum 2006;54(1):158–68.
[67] Strand V, Kavanaugh AF. The role of interleukin-1 in bone resorption in rheumatoid arthritis. Rheumatology (Oxford) 2004;43(Suppl 3):iii10–6.
[68] Joosten LA, Helsen MM, van de Loo FA, et al. Anticytokine treatment of established type II collagen-induced arthritis in DBA/1 mice. A comparative study using anti-TNF alpha, anti-IL-1 alpha/beta, and IL-1Ra. Arthritis Rheum 1996;39(5):797–809.
[69] Maini RN, Breedveld FC, Kalden JR, et al. Sustained improvement over two years in physical function, structural damage, and signs and symptoms among patients with rheumatoid arthritis treated with infliximab and methotrexate. Arthritis Rheum 2004;50(4):1051–65.
[70] Pincus T, Yazici Y, Sokka T, et al. Methotrexate as the "anchor drug" for the treatment of early rheumatoid arthritis. Clin Exp Rheumatol 2003;21(5)(Suppl 31)S179–85.
[71] Seitz M, Zwicker M, Loetscher P. Effects of methotrexate on differentiation of monocytes and production of cytokine inhibitors by monocytes. Arthritis Rheum 1998;41(11):2032–8.
[72] Li P, Schwarz EM, O'Keefe RJ, et al. RANK signaling is not required for TNFalpha-mediated increase in CD11(hi) osteoclast precursors but is essential for mature osteoclast formation in TNFalpha-mediated inflammatory arthritis. J Bone Miner Res 2004;19(2):207–13.
[73] Goldring SR. Bone and joint destruction in rheumatoid arthritis: what is really happening? J Rheumatol Suppl 2002;65:44–8.
[74] Stanton H, Rogerson FM, East CJ, et al. ADAMTS5 is the major aggrecanase in mouse cartilage in vivo and in vitro. Nature 2005;434(7033):648–52.
[75] Glasson SS, Askew R, Sheppard B, et al. Deletion of active ADAMTS5 prevents cartilage degradation in a murine model of osteoarthritis. Nature 2005;434(7033):644–8.
[76] Tanaka S, Nakamura K, Takahasi N, et al. Role of RANKL in physiological and pathological bone resorption and therapeutics targeting the RANKL-RANK signaling system. Immunol Rev 2005;208:30–49.
[77] Bekker PJ, Holloway DL, Rasmussen AS, et al. A single-dose placebo-controlled study of AMG 162, a fully human monoclonal antibody to RANKL, in postmenopausal women. J Bone Miner Res 2004;19(7):1059–66.
[78] McClung MR, Lewiecki EM, Cohen SB, et al. Denosumab in postmenopausal women with low bone mineral density. N Engl J Med 2006;354(8):821–31.
[79] Juji T, Hertz M, Aoki K, et al. A novel therapeutic vaccine approach, targeting RANKL, prevents bone destruction in bone-related disorders. J Bone Miner Metab 2002;20(5):266–8.
[80] Russell RG, Rogers MJ. Bisphosphonates: from the laboratory to the clinic and back again. Bone 1999;25(1):97–106.
[81] Green JR. Bisphosphonates: preclinical review. Oncologist 2004;9(Suppl 4):3–13.
[82] Osterman T, Kippo K, Lauren L, et al. Effect of clodronate on established collagen-induced arthritis in rats. Inflamm Res 1995;44(6):258–63.

[83] Osterman T, Kippo K, Lauren L, Pasanen I, Hannuniemi R, Sellman R. A comparison of clodronate and indomethacin in the treatment of adjuvant arthritis. Inflamm Res 1997; 46(3):79–85.

[84] Kinne RW, Schmidt-Weber CB, Hoppe R, et al. Long-term amelioration of rat adjuvant arthritis following systemic elimination of macrophages by clodronate-containing liposomes. Arthritis Rheum 1995;38(12):1777–90.

[85] Kinne RW, Schmidt CB, Buchner E, et al. Treatment of rat arthritides with clodronate-containing liposomes. Scand J Rheumatol Suppl 1995;101:91–7.

[86] Romas E. Bone loss in inflammatory arthritis: mechanisms and therapeutic approaches with bisphosphonates. Best Pract Res Clin Rheumatol 2005;19(6):1065–79.

[87] Jarrett S, Conaghan PG, Sloan VS, et al. Preliminary evidence for a structural benefit of the new bisphosphonate zoledronic acid in early rheumatoid arthritis. Arthritis Rheum 2006; 54(5):1410–4.

[88] Sharp JT, Van Der Heijde D, Boers M, et al. Repair of erosions in rheumatoid arthritis does occur. Results from 2 studies by the OMERACT Subcommittee on Healing of Erosions. J Rheumatol 2003;30(5):1102–7.

[89] Martin TJ, Sims NA. Osteoclast-derived activity in the coupling of bone formation to resorption. Trends Mol Med 2005;11(2):76–81.

[90] Gilbert LC, Rubin J, Nanes MS. The p55 TNF receptor mediates TNF inhibition of osteoblast differentiation independently of apoptosis. Am J Physiol Endocrinol Metab 2005; 288(5):E1011–8.

[91] Gilbert L, He X, Farmer P, et al. Expression of the osteoblast differentiation factor RUNX2 (Cbfa1/AML3/Pebp2alpha A) is inhibited by tumor necrosis factor-alpha. J Biol Chem 2002;277(4):2695–701.

[92] Hodsman AB, Bauer DC, Dempster DW, et al. Parathyroid hormone and teriparatide for the treatment of osteoporosis: a review of the evidence and suggested guidelines for its use. Endocr Rev 2005;26(5):688–703.

[93] Redlich K, Gortz B, Hayer S, et al. Repair of local bone erosions and reversal of systemic bone loss upon therapy with anti-tumor necrosis factor in combination with osteoprotegerin or parathyroid hormone in tumor necrosis factor-mediated arthritis. Am J Pathol 2004; 164(2):543–55.

[94] Schett G, Middleton S, Bolon B, et al. Additive bone-protective effects of anabolic treatment when used in conjunction with RANKL and tumor necrosis factor inhibition in two rat arthritis models. Arthritis Rheum 2005;52(5):1604–11.

[95] Sugiyama T, Tanaka H, Kawai S. Effects of parathyroid hormone and alendronate alone or in combination in osteoporosis. N Engl J Med 2004;350(2):189–92 [author reply 189–92].

[96] Higashida J, Wun T, Schmidt S, et al. Safety and efficacy of rituximab in patients with rheumatoid arthritis refractory to disease modifying antirheumatic drugs and anti-tumor necrosis factor-alpha treatment. J Rheumatol 2005;32(11):2109–15.

[97] Genovese MC, Becker JC, Schiff M, et al. Abatacept for rheumatoid arthritis refractory to tumor necrosis factor alpha inhibition. N Engl J Med 2005;353(11):1114–23.

[98] Goldring SR, Gravallese EM. Bisphosphonates: environmental protection for the joint? Arthritis Rheum 2004;50(7):2044–7.

[99] Farrugia MC, Summerlin DJ, Krowiak E, et al. Osteonecrosis of the mandible or maxilla associated with the use of new generation bisphosphonates. Laryngoscope 2006;116(1): 115–20.

ELSEVIER
SAUNDERS

Rheum Dis Clin N Am 32 (2006) 775–780

RHEUMATIC
DISEASE CLINICS
OF NORTH AMERICA

Index

Note: Page numbers of article titles are in **boldface** type.

0889-857X/06/$ - see front matter © 2006 Elsevier Inc. All rights reserved.
doi:10.1016/S0889-857X(06)00082-2

rheumatic.theclinics.com

United States Postal Service
Statement of Ownership, Management, and Circulation

1. Publication Title	2. Publication Number	3. Filing Date
Rheumatic Disease Clinics of North America	0 0 6 - 2 7 2	9/15/06

4. Issue Frequency	5. Number of Issues Published Annually	6. Annual Subscription Price
Feb, May, Aug, Nov	4	$190.00

7. Complete Mailing Address of Known Office of Publication (Not printer) (Street, city, county, state, and ZIP+4)

Elsevier, Inc.
360 Park Avenue South
New York, NY 10010-1710

Contact Person
Sarah Carmichael
Telephone
(215) 239-3681

8. Complete Mailing Address of Headquarters or General Business Office of Publisher (Not printer)

Elsevier, Inc., 360 Park Avenue South, New York, NY 10010-1710

9. Full Names and Complete Mailing Addresses of Publisher, Editor, and Managing Editor (Do not leave blank)

Publisher (Name and complete mailing address)

John Schrefer, Elsevier, Inc., 1600 John F. Kennedy Blvd., Suite 1800, Philadelphia, PA 19103-2899

Editor (Name and complete mailing address)

Rachel Glover, Elsevier, Inc., 1600 John F. Kennedy Blvd., Suite 1300, Philadelphia, PA 19103-2899

Managing Editor (Name and complete mailing address)

Catherine Bewick, Elsevier, Inc., 1600 John F. Kennedy Blvd., Suite 1800, Philadelphia, PA 19103-2899

10. Owner (Do not leave blank. If the publication is owned by a corporation, give the name and address of the corporation immediately followed by the names and addresses of all stockholders owning or holding 1 percent or more of the total amount of stock. If not owned by a corporation, give the names and addresses of the individual owners. If owned by a partnership or other unincorporated firm, give its name and address as well as those of each individual owner. If the publication is published by a nonprofit organization, give its name and address.)

Full Name	Complete Mailing Address
Wholly owned subsidiary of	4520 East-West Highway
Reed/Elsevier, US Holdings	Bethesda, MD 20814

11. Known Bondholders, Mortgagees, and Other Security Holders Owning or Holding 1 Percent or More of Total Amount of Bonds, Mortgages, or Other Securities. If none, check box ▶ None

Full Name	Complete Mailing Address
N/A	

12. Tax Status (For completion by nonprofit organizations authorized to mail at nonprofit rates) (Check one)
The purpose, function, and nonprofit status of this organization and the exempt status for federal income tax purposes:
☐ Has Not Changed During Preceding 12 Months
☐ Has Changed During Preceding 12 Months (Publisher must submit explanation of change with this statement)

(See Instructions on Reverse)

PS Form 3526, October 1999

13. Publication Title	14. Issue Date for Circulation Data Below
Rheumatic Disease Clinics of North America	August, 2006

15.	Extent and Nature of Circulation	Average No. Copies Each Issue During Preceding 12 Months	No. Copies of Single Issue Published Nearest to Filing Date
a.	Total Number of Copies (Net press run)	2,775	2,600
b. Paid and/or Requested Circulation	(1) Paid/Requested Outside-County Mail Subscriptions Stated on Form 3541. (Include advertiser's proof and exchange copies)	1,128	1,013
	(2) Paid In-County Subscriptions Stated on Form 3541 (Include advertiser's proof and exchange copies)		
	(3) Sales Through Dealers and Carriers, Street Vendors, Counter Sales, and Other Non-USPS Paid Distribution	719	688
	(4) Other Classes Mailed Through the USPS		
c.	Total Paid and/or Requested Circulation [Sum of 15b. (1), (2), (3), and (4)] ▶	1,847	1,701
d. Free Distribution by Mail (Samples, complimentary, and other free)	(1) Outside-County as Stated on Form 3541	113	103
	(2) In-County as Stated on Form 3541		
	(3) Other Classes Mailed Through the USPS		
e.	Free Distribution Outside the Mail (Carriers or other means)		
f.	Total Free Distribution (Sum of 15d. and 15e.) ▶	113	103
g.	Total Distribution (Sum of 15c. and 15f.) ▶	1,960	1,804
h.	Copies not Distributed	815	796
i.	Total (Sum of 15g. and h.) ▶	2,775	2,600
j.	Percent Paid and/or Requested Circulation (15c. divided by 15g. times 100)	94.23%	94.29%

16. Publication of Statement of Ownership
☒ Publication required. Will be printed in the November 2006 issue of this publication. ☐ Publication not required.

17. Signature and Title of Editor, Publisher, Business Manager, or Owner   Date

[signature]
Joseph Frances - Executive Director of Subscription Services   9/15/06

I certify that all information furnished on this form is true and complete. I understand that anyone who furnishes false or misleading information on this form or who omits material or information requested on the form may be subject to criminal sanctions (including fines and imprisonment) and/or civil sanctions (including civil penalties).

Instructions to Publishers

1. Complete and file one copy of this form with your postmaster annually on or before October 1. Keep a copy of the completed form for your records.
2. In cases where the stockholder or security holder is a trustee, include in items 10 and 11 the name of the person or corporation for whom the trustee is acting. Also include the names and addresses of individuals who are stockholders who own or hold 1 percent or more of the total amount of bonds, mortgages, or other securities of the publishing corporation. In item 11, if none, check the box. Use blank sheets if more space is required.
3. Be sure to furnish all circulation information called for in item 15. Free circulation must be shown in items 15d, e, and f.
4. Item 15h., Copies not Distributed, must include (1) newsstand copies originally stated on Form 3541, and returned to the publisher, (2) estimated returns from news agents, and (3) copies for office use, leftovers, spoiled, and all other copies not distributed.
5. If the publication had Periodicals authorization as a general or requester publication, this Statement of Ownership, Management, and Circulation must be published; it must be printed in any issue in October or, if the publication is not published during October, the first issue printed after October.
6. In item 16, indicate the date of the issue in which this Statement of Ownership will be published.
7. Item 17 must be signed.
Failure to file or publish a statement of ownership may lead to suspension of Periodicals authorization.

PS Form 3526, October 1999 (Reverse)

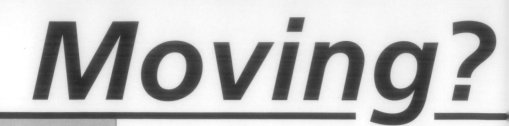

Moving?

Make sure your subscription moves with you!

To notify us of your new address, find your **Clinics Account Number** (located on your mailing label above your name), and contact customer service at:

E-mail: elspcs@elsevier.com

800-654-2452 (subscribers in the U.S. & Canada)
407-345-4000 (subscribers outside of the U.S. & Canada)

Fax number: 407-363-9661

Elsevier Periodicals Customer Service
6277 Sea Harbor Drive
Orlando, FL 32887-4800

*To ensure uninterrupted delivery of your subscription, please notify us at least 4 weeks in advance of move.

ELSEVIER